Organic Body Care

How to Make Natural Body Scrubs, Body Butters, and Bath Bombs

Contents

Part 1: Body Scrubs

The Ultimate DIY Guide on How to Make Your Own Natural Body Scrubs, Including Simple and Organic Recipes

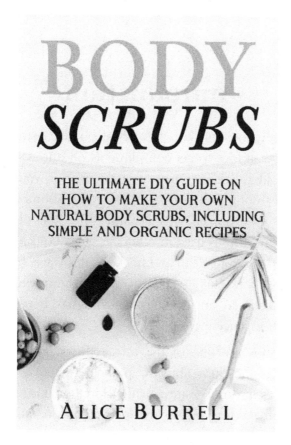

Introduction

Having healthy, radiant skin goes far beyond its aesthetic aspects. Naturally, we all love to get compliments on our skin, especially as we get older, and we aim to maintain our youthful looks. However, a smooth, plump skin texture also shows that you are taking care of yourself, inside and out. This boosts your confidence and instills trust in others as well. To achieve all this, our skin must be kept clean and healthy - this is where exfoliation plays a huge part. This essential routine of removing dead skin cells dates back to ancient Egypt - and has been present in various cultures since then.

Body scrubs are one of the most efficient ways of manual exfoliation as they use abrasive particles that can unclog the deepest pores. From moisturizing the skin to making it healthier - scrubbing off its dead layers provides your skin with numerous other benefits. Every time you exfoliate, you are revitalizing your skin, but you are also replenishing your overall health and vitality. With the right ingredients and technique, body scrubbing can provide you with a complete and relaxing spa experience in the comfort of your own home.

Now, if you want to take advantage of all the benefits that body scrubs can provide, you will need to learn how to make your own. In this book, you will receive comprehensive and practical guidance on making simple, organic body scrubs from everyday ingredients. Doing this will allow you to find effective yet inexpensive solutions to improve your skin tone and health. More importantly, you will learn how to make customized exfoliants that will fit the present needs of your skin.

If you don't have experience using body scrubs, you may find the prospect of making them even more challenging. Fortunately, you won't have to worry about figuring out complicated measurements or preparation methods. From the hands-on instructions to the benefits of each recipe, you'll find everything you need in this book. Furthermore, all the recipes use ingredients you probably already have in your pantry. So, anytime you need some pampering, you can just make a batch of body scrubs and enjoy a relaxing experience.

Like any beauty product, learning how to use body scrubs takes some trial and error. Still, if you can use homemade, organic products, you will have far better chances of succeeding. No one knows your body and skin better than you do. You are the one who can see the subtle changes in your skin tone and texture, and therefore you are the one who can satisfy all its needs. Remember, these often change due to both internal and external factors. While the internal issues can be remedied through a healthier diet and lifestyle, this book will teach you how to keep your skin healthy from the outside via homemade body scrubs. If you are ready to learn how to make products to pamper your skin in the best way possible, don't hesitate to keep reading.

Chapter 1: Body Scrubs— Basics

Your skin has the amazing ability to renew itself and provide you with protection from the outside elements. Skin cells die during this regeneration process and allow the new ones to execute their roles. While shedding dead skin happens naturally, it's usually a very long process influenced by your lifestyle and environment. Meanwhile, these dead cells remain on top of your skin, creating a buildup that will make your skin look dry and lifeless. Exfoliating with body scrubs can help your skin look healthier and feel smooth. Due to their unique texture, these products encourage the shedding of those unnecessary layers, refining the skin's surface a lot more quickly than would happen naturally.

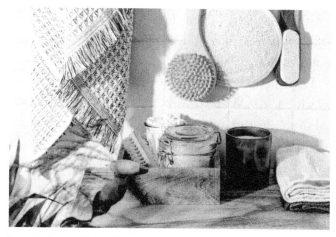

By taking away the dead skin cells, body scrubs unclog your pores, significantly decreasing the risk of blemishes, ingrown hairs, and infections. Buffing the skin in this manner is particularly important if you regularly wax or shave, as these processes open hair follicles, essentially creating small traps for the debris on your skin. Body scrubbing renews your body, and pampering yourself encourages self-love as well. Taking care of yourself leaves you with polished and smooth skin, but it also represents a wonderful chance to escape the day-to-day stresses. It's a treatment that you deserve and need – because feeling refreshed means being empowered to take on new challenges in life!

History of Body Scrubs

While nowadays you can read about it online more and more, skin exfoliation isn't a new beauty routine. Records show that ancient Egyptians used various methods to keep their skin healthy and glowing, including body scrubs. By combining natural materials with a particle-like texture with fragrant essential oils, they could prevent their skin from becoming dry and flaky, despite their scorching heat. Not only that, but their formulas had a very effective anti-aging effect as well. However, the Egyptians were not the only ones using body scrubs. Historical evidence shows that similar exfoliation techniques were used in numerous other cultures for thousands of years. In Europe, during the Middle Ages, people often made body scrubs from grapeseed and tartaric acid. Widespread use of exfoliation has been recorded in the history of China as well, under the three-century-long rule of the Qing Dynasty. All these cultures recognize the importance of pampering one's skin with natural ingredients and giving it a chance to breathe and regenerate itself.

How to Apply Body Scrubs

If you haven't used a particular body scrub before, it's a good idea to do a small patch test to see how your skin reacts to the formula. The skin on your body isn't as delicate as the skin on your face, although it can still be sensitive to a new ingredient, so it doesn't hurt to take the necessary precautions. Apply a tiny dollop on your hand, massage it in with a circular motion, wash it off, and wait for any reaction. If you notice any redness or itching on that particular area within 48 hours, don't apply the scrub to the rest of your body. If not, the product is safe to use, and you can proceed with the exfoliation.

Before starting to exfoliate, you will need to prepare your skin for the process. A body scrub will need to enter your pores and clean your skin properly. Fortunately, this preparation process does not entail any complicated setup. All it takes is for you to take a long shower or bath in moderately warm water, and the scrub of your choice will be able to work its magic. Wet, warm skin will allow you to evenly distribute the formula on its surface, including the open pores. Warm water is also the perfect way to relax your mind and body, thus kicking off that perfect spa-like experience. Make sure you shampoo as well before applying the body scrub as your skin may be too sensitive to wash afterward. Also, if you want to apply a moisturizing body scrub with essential oils, washing them off will defeat their purpose.

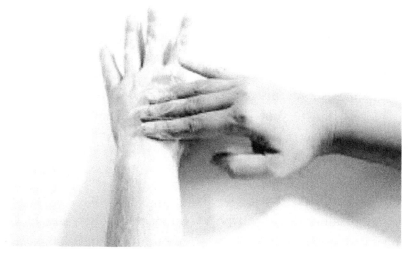

Once you have rinsed yourself after the shower or bath you have taken, choose your scrub and apply a generous amount of it onto your still-wet skin. Distribute each dollop by massaging it gently into your skin. It's recommended to begin with your torso and move towards your limbs while working in circular movements, taking about 30 seconds per area. While the rest can be done standing up, when you get to your feet, you will need to sit down to better access them and avoid slipping and hurting yourself.

While simply applying it with your hands can have nice effects, if you want the exfoliant to have an even greater and long-lasting impact, you will need to work it into your skin with an exfoliating body mitt or brush. These will help you get the scrub into all of your pores and clean them more thoroughly without being too harsh to your skin. When you have finished massaging your body and you're getting to your limbs, stop the circular motion and switch to single-line strokes. Doing this backward toward your heart will finish the revitalizing process by improving circulation in your limbs.

Once you are satisfied that the exfoliant has been distributed and worked evenly throughout your body, you can rinse it off with lukewarm water. If you have taken a bath beforehand, you may do this in the remaining bathwater, but running water is more effective in washing off the scrub particles, so it's best to take a quick shower instead. When doing this, make sure you go over every part of your body to help the water wash everything away. When no particles remain, you can turn off the water and pat yourself dry. Avoid rubbing yourself dry with a towel because this will remove the moisturizing effect of the product. Already, your skin will feel much smoother, although it may feel a little dry, depending on what type of exfoliant you have used. To enhance the softness of your skin, moisturize with a lotion that matches your skin type after each scrubbing.

While shaving right afterward may cause some irritation, it's also the best time to get rid of that unwanted hair as well. Remember, your pores are open and cleaned, making hair removal much easier and the care afterward less complicated. However, if you choose to shave after scrubbing, make sure you apply a generous amount of moisturizing lotion after towel drying yourself gently.

If you notice any type of irritation while applying a patch test without any adverse effects while the scrub is being applied, stop working it into the rest of your body, and wash it off immediately. You shouldn't use this type of exfoliant again, nor should you use any in general if you have any open wounds, eczema, or burns (even sunburn). People with severe acne should only use body scrubs after consulting with a dermatologist who can determine which type of products will be safe for them to use.

Precautions to Take After Exfoliation

Even though body scrubbing is great to keep your skin in great condition, this is only possible if you take some other precautions. Here are some of the things you should avoid doing after scrubbing:

- **Sunbathing:** Exposing your skin to sunlight after being scrubbed is not a good idea. Your skin has less protection against the harmful effects of the sun and is also more sensitive, which means that you can easily end up with sunburns.

- **Further Exfoliation:** If you have chosen the proper application method, the body scrub should have done its job in exfoliating your skin. Applying another method right after scrubbing will cause irritation. If you feel that your skin hasn't been exfoliated enough, wait at least two days before continuing the process.

- **Sauna:** While warm water is necessary to prep your skin for exfoliation, continuing to expose yourself to it after using a body scrub dries out the skin and can cause darker blotches to appear. For this reason, it's better to avoid using a steam room or sauna immediately after scrubbing.

- **Waxing:** Shaving may be permitted after scrubbing, but waxing is definitely a no-no. Waxing alone can cause severe irritation to your skin, and combining it with mechanical exfoliation may even result in minor injuries.

How Often Should You Exfoliate?

Since exfoliation involves mechanically working the scrub into the skin, it can damage your skin's surface layers if done too often. No matter how moisturizing its formula is, it has to contain an abrasive particle to function as a deep cleanser. Furthermore, once removed, it will take some time for the dead skin cells to build up again, so there is no need to make body scrubbing part of your everyday routine like you do with moisturizing. Typically, it's not recommended to exfoliate your skin more than twice a week. If your skin feels particularly dry, try applying a rich lotion instead – a scrub would probably only make it dryer. If this happens, avoid using body scrubs for a while until your skin improves. Oily skin often requires more frequent exfoliation, but you still don't want to overdo it. Removing the oil too often will make your skin produce even more sebum, clogging your pores and leading to more blemishes.

Some skin types require less frequent exfoliation, and some have ever-changing needs. Make sure you pay attention to your skin, especially when seasons are changing or if you are experiencing a stressful period in your life. Doing this will allow you to react swiftly to any change in your skin tone by applying the product that will restore its balance. If you haven't used body scrubs before, it may take time for you to get totally attuned to your skin's needs, and you will probably make some mistakes as you learn. Due to their natural formula, applying the scrub one or two times usually won't have any serious consequences, but it will help you learn what your skin really needs. People with darker skin tones are also warned against overly aggressive and frequent scrubbing because it may lead to the appearance of darker or lighter areas that will dry out more quickly than the rest of the body.

Benefits of Body Scrubbing

Regular body scrubbing should be part of everyone's self-care routine and for several reasons. Exfoliating products contain an abrasive ingredient that mechanically removes all the debris from the surface of your skin, allowing you to clean your body more thoroughly. Clean skin is always easier to keep healthy, especially if you shave regularly. As mentioned before, during exfoliation, all the debris is removed from your pores, so when you shave, you won't end up with ingrown hair and razor bumps caused by clogged pores. Apart from being a nuisance, razor bumps and ingrown hair can end up causing serious infections that can spread beyond your skin and result in other health complications as well.

Your skin's natural shedding ability works quite slowly to begin with, and it can also be affected by numerous factors. A sudden change in environment can slow the process down even more, as does aging. As you get older, the less your skin will shed, which means you will require more frequent exfoliation. At the same time, older skin loses its ability to retain moisture, and you will need all the hydration you can get, including that which comes from essential oils in a body scrub. Since the abrasive particles need to be bound together in a solid mass, body scrubs also contain a wet ingredient which typically has a moisturizing effect. Regardless of your skin type, keeping it hydrated is another requirement for its health. Certain cleansing products can have very drying effects, especially if they aren't suitable for your skin type. Wearing a lot of makeup on your face and body irritates the skin and clogs the pores, which need the type of deep cleansing only exfoliating with body scrubs can provide.

Both overly cold and hot weather can be quite damaging for your skin, and not just because of dehydration. Prolonged exposure to extreme elements leads to premature aging, discoloration, and the skin's decreased ability to protect you from infections. Body scrubs can provide the skin with all the nutrients it needs to keep itself and your body healthy. It may take some time to figure out what your body needs, but once you do, you will be able to use them in your own homemade products as well. In addition to making the skin absorb the nutrients through open pores during scrubbing, exfoliation also facilitates further hydration. Not only will this work right after body scrubbing, but without those dead skin cells in the way, the moisturizer you apply in your everyday skincare will get right where it needs to be.

Body scrubs have a smoothing effect which not only improves the appearance of dry or blemish-prone skin, but it's even more effective on older skin. With the proper type of moisturizing agents, you can make your skin feel much younger and even slow down the aging process. However, it's worth mentioning that younger skin can look more aged than it really is without proper care. If your skin is on the dry side, and you don't moisturize or exfoliate regularly, eventually, its surface becomes flaky and lifeless. Even one good scrubbing can make your skin look much smoother and more even-textured.

If you have combination skin and one method of exfoliation doesn't work for your entire body, feel free to apply several mechanical exfoliation techniques. For example, if your face is more sensitive, but you still want to use the same product that you've used on your body, you can always apply it gently by lightly tapping with a face cloth. Suppose you feel your skin requires deeper exfoliation in some areas of your body. In that case, you can use a loofah there or do a dry skin brushing beforehand.

If you aren't used to pampering yourself in this way, it may be a curious experience initially, but once you make scrubbing a regular part of your beauty routine, you will never stop doing it. After all, who wouldn't want to have radiant, perfectly clean skin that retains moisture and ages at a much slower rate?

Why Use Homemade Body Scrubs?

While there are numerous other exfoliation methods, scrubs are clearly more advantageous than most of them. One of their biggest perks is that everyone can make them at home without any qualifications. These DIY exfoliants only consist of a few natural, easily available ingredients that you can combine to suit your needs. Essentially, the only two things you will have to consider are the grit and the level of hydration. The grit refers to the size of the particles used and determines the effectiveness of the exfoliation. Here it's important to note that you may need different types of grit at different times. When your skin feels drier, you need a finer grit. If it's more oily, feel free to use larger particles next time. Also, you should avoid using heavier grit too often as this can lead to skin irritation. The hydration level is adjusted by the number of moist agents, which are typically essential oils. This is particularly helpful for people with overly sensitive skin who can add only very fine particles, allowing for very gentle scrubbing. Similarly, if you have dry or oily skin, you can add more or less moisturizing ingredients to your liking. You can even alter the particular product with seasonal changes to always provide your skin with everything it needs to stay healthy and glowing.

Apart from the active exfoliant, commercial body scrubs often contain additional ingredients that may be too harsh to apply to your skin. Even if your skin isn't too delicate, applying chemicals onto your skin isn't the healthiest choice, especially in these modern times when we are surrounded by pollution everywhere we go. By making the body scrubs from scratch, you are in control of the entire process. You are free to use organic ingredients and avoid harsh and potentially harmful chemicals.

Applying a body scrub at home could provide you with the full spa experience without paying for costly services. However, ready-made commercial products containing quality ingredients can still be quite expensive. Therefore, making organic body scrubs is not only a much healthier alternative, but it's definitely budget-friendly as well. You probably already have some of these ingredients in your home (like sugar, oats, or coffee) and use them for other purposes. The ones you may not have (like essential oils) are still relatively inexpensive - yet they will still exfoliate your skin very efficiently. Apart from being less expensive than a spa treatment, homemade body scrubs are also far more convenient. After learning how to make the ones that suit your skin type the best, you will be able to whip up a batch anytime you feel your skin could use some pampering.

While the most popular commercial body scrubs are typically sugar or salt-based, there is a wide variety of other exfoliating agents you can use. Coffee grounds or oats are also great ingredients that provide excellent mechanical exfoliation effects yet are widely available and inexpensive. Just make sure the ones you use are suitable for your specific skin type. This may take some time to determine, but the beauty of using organic products lies exactly in that they allow you to do that. Fewer chemicals mean less chance of skin irritation, allergies, or any other adverse reaction. The overall benefits you can gain from experimenting with DIY body scrubs override most risks. In the meantime, you get to learn so much about your skin and body. Plus, you will have a relaxing experience when using the scrubs you have made yourself. More information about particular homemade body scrubs will be detailed in the following chapters.

Chapter 2: Choosing Your Exfoliant

Everybody scrub needs three quintessential elements: the exfoliants, the carrier oils, and the essential oils. These simple ingredients are present in most store-bought scrubs, along with preservatives, coloring, soap, and even artificial fragrance. However, for a DIY product at home, you only have to mix together the three main components depending on your personal needs and preferences. In addition to the fact that most recipes are all the same for the main type of ingredients, the products you need for them are common household items that you may use daily. This simplicity makes DIY body scrubs simple, inexpensive, and easy to tailor to anyone's skin.

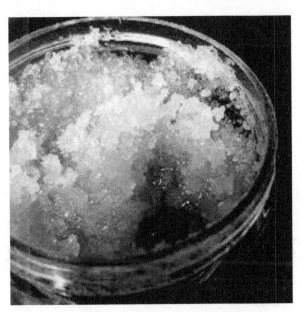

The exfoliant is the ingredient that scrubs away all the dead cells from the skin's surface, which means choosing the right one is paramount for the desired effect. An exfoliant has to have a particle-like consistency - which, when it comes in contact with skin, will scrape its surface and go deep into the pores. The most common exfoliants in body scrubs are sugar, salt, ground coffee, oatmeal, grains, ground herbal seeds, and groundnuts. While it's typical for one exfoliant to be added at a time, if needed, they can be combined as well.

The carrier oil is added to hold the mixture into one spreadable mass. Furthermore, since the exfoliants are usually dry ingredients, you wouldn't be able to massage them into your skin in their natural state. The oils make the scrub go on smoothly and without scratching your skin. Most commercial scrub manufacturers combine multiple oils to reach the perfect consistency for the product to become marketable. Fortunately, when making homemade scrubs, the only thing you will have to worry about is what feels good on your skin. Because they are also used in many kitchens, olive, coconut, sunflower, and grapeseed oils probably have the most widespread usage in body scrubs. Apart from these, some recipes may use sesame, jojoba, walnut, or sweet almond oils. Keep in mind that some ingredients may not be suitable for people with severe food allergies.

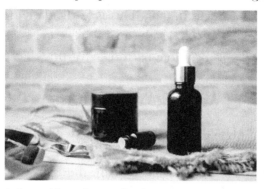

While a scrub could work just fine just as a deep cleanser with the first two ingredients, if you want to step up the experience, you can also mix some essential oils into your scrub. It will be up to you whether you do it to make the mixture more fragrant, help you relax while applying, moisturize your skin, or help it heal and rejuvenate. The choice of oils you can use is almost limitless - you will only have to find the ones that suit your skin best. Please note that you should avoid using certain types of oils if you are pregnant.

Some homemade scrub recipes contain soap as well, even though this is typically added as a stabilizing agent and doesn't have any impact on your skin. It's usually used alongside fine particle exfoliants that can be used up to 2-3 times a week as they aren't as harsh on the skin. Others may prefer adding preservatives as well. That being said, the beauty of homemade scrubs lies in their simplicity and fast preparation methods, so there is hardly a need to store them too long. Typically, organic scrubs can be stored for at least a couple of days without worrying about them spoiling too quickly. The exfoliants alone can last for months, but the usability of your scrub depends on the ingredients as well. The essential oils are safe to use for up to a couple of years, while the other components have a shelf life depending on their nature and storage temperatures. Keep in mind that higher temperatures and humidity levels facilitate the growth of bacteria, so you will need to keep your exfoliants in a colder and drier environment. This is particularly true if sugar is used as an exfoliant alongside an edible carrier because these types of ingredients promote bacterial growth.

Sugar Scrubs

If you have skin that's either normal or just a little bit on the drier side but is often sensitive, you will benefit from sugar scrubs. Since its particles are smaller than the grit other exfoliants provide, sugar is one of the gentlest exfoliants. This makes it safe to use all over your body, including your face. Sugar is also one of the ingredients almost everyone has in their pantry, so you can make a budget-friendly scrub anytime you want to. For example, if you plan to shave, you will definitely need to exfoliate beforehand. Doing it with a sugar scrub won't make your skin overly sensitive, so you can safely shave afterward. By massaging sugar into the body areas you will shave later, you open up your follicles and unclog all the pores. This is important to facilitate the shaving process and prevent ingrown hairs and razor bumps.

Besides chemical exfoliation, the natural way, applying sugar scrubs to your skin has numerous other advantages. Like their salty counterparts, sugar scrubs also allow your skin to retain more moisture and contain elements that help skin regeneration by accelerating cell growth. Apart from making your skin smoother, this will also ensure that your skin stays healthy and able to defend itself from toxins. By gently removing the dead cells that are making your skin look flaky, lifeless, and much older, sugar scrubs can brighten your entire appearance. This makes sugar one of the most natural anti-aging agents you can safely apply to your skin.

While having a long warm bath or shower before exfoliating is recommended, sometimes you just don't have that much time to complete this pampering ritual. Fortunately, sugar dissolves much faster than any other exfoliant, so it only needs your skin to be slightly wet before application. You can just take a quick shower, apply the scrub all over your body, and rinse it off when finished.

If you want to share the benefits of your DIY body scrubs and gift them to your family and friends but aren't sure which type would suit them best, a sugar scrub is the safest choice. Sugar exfoliants are mild enough to be applied safely on the most sensitive skin types, and at the same time, very effective in polishing the skin. Just make sure you prepare the scrubs from natural sugars rich in beneficial minerals and glycolic acid - and without an ingredient, the recipient might be allergic to them.

Salt Scrubs

Salt scrubs can be the perfect option if you have particularly oily skin or haven't exfoliated in a while. Salts, as exfoliants, tend to be abrasive on the skin, which means they are more effective in unclogging your pores, helping to keep your skin healthy, despite the amount of sebum it produces. However, due to their rather aggressive nature, salts should never be applied to your face - or any areas of your body with overly sensitive skin.

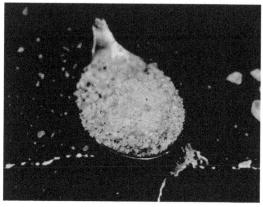

https://unsplash.com/photos/pink-powder-on-black-frying-pan-CYreeF3l7CY

The longer you wait between scrubbings, the more extensive the cell buildup will be on your skin. Apart from being unhygienic, this will also cause your skin to look hardened and patchy. On certain parts of your body, over time, these layers become thicker and thicker, ultimately forming calluses. Other exfoliants may not remove the thickened skin from your heels, knees, and elbows, but salts will deal with this issue very effectively. Depending on how deep the calluses are, removing them may take some time. However, the application of salt scrubs can help reveal the renewed skin that's hiding underneath.

For the best exfoliation results, these types of scrubs should be applied by massaging them gently into the skin for about 30 seconds per area until the salt granules dissolve. This will also help the salt strip the debris from the surface, and once washed off, your skin will shine from becoming healthy instead of shining due to the excess oils. Removing dead cells alone promotes the growth of new ones and allows for deeper moisturization. Using salt scrubs can make your skin absorb any lotion you are using much faster and more effectively. Massaging an abrasive substance like salt into your skin also improves its circulation, further stimulating your skin's regenerative abilities. After only a couple of applications, your skin will be much firmer and rejuvenated.

Not only are salts natural humectants and will keep your skin free of oils, but they also have antibacterial properties. Reducing the number of bacteria on your skin is crucial to prevent blemishes, especially if you are prone to having frequent bouts of them. If you already have acne on your skin, applying salt scrubs on any problematic area (except for your face) will effectively reduce inflammation. It may alleviate other symptoms like itching and pain as well. However, with this type of skin, it's better to apply it gently and let your skin soak it up for a couple of minutes rather than rubbing it in aggressively. Doing the latter will irritate your skin, which will make it produce even more oils, making the entire process counterproductive.

Coffee Scrubs

In their natural form, ground coffee particles can cleanse your skin of any debris and help it fight off toxins and bacteria. Combined with sugars and essential oils, coffee-based exfoliants can do much more than that. Coffee will make your skin soak up the oils faster, so you won't have to wait until your skin gets hydrated. The effects will be visible as soon as you wash the scrub off and pat yourself dry.

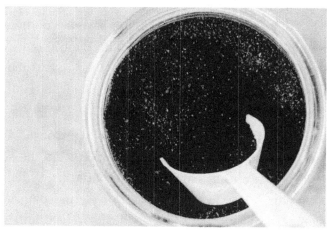

https://unsplash.com/photos/white-table-spoon-on-coffee-chymerU7QFI

Coffee scrubs are usually recommended to those who want to tighten their skin by eliminating cellulite. Caffeine simply redirects blood flow from the puffy surface of the skin to the still-developing cells underneath. As the blood flows away, the skin appears tighter and can regenerate itself very quickly. In fact, if you are fighting stubborn cellulite, coffee grounds are probably one of the most effective solutions for this problem. Considering its budget-friendly pricing, exfoliation with coffee is also one of the most cost-effective skin tightening treatments you can give yourself. Of course, there are lots of caffeine-based commercial anti-cellulite treatments as well. However, an organic product is always a healthier alternative to free yourself of the toxins accumulated in your cellulite. Coffee exfoliants reduce the need for unnecessary chemicals on your skin that often clog your pores and accelerate your skin's aging process.

The same way a cup of coffee can energize your mind by boosting brain circulation, the application of caffeine on the skin stimulates capillary circulation. Combined with fast, circular movements as you apply coffee scrub the body, this exfoliant promotes blood flow to all your skin cells. Improved circulation leads to faster skin cell regeneration and a smooth surface. Caffeine can also act as a powerful antioxidant, reducing inflammation. In smaller quantities, it can be applied around your eyes to reduce swelling and diminish the puffiness and discoloration in the under-eye region. The same way it reduces cellulite, a coffee exfoliant can also smoothen out wrinkles and other visible effects of aging, significantly changing your skin's texture.

By removing the dead skin, coffee scrubs exfoliate the skin and repair its structure. Inadequate protection from the sun and prolonged exposure to its harmful UV rays can leave their mark on your skin. To help combat long-term damage like hyperpigmentation, and sunspots, exfoliate with a coffee scrub once a week. After only a couple of applications, your skin tone will become even and radiant. Even if the skin is irritated from recent sun exposure, a gently applied coffee exfoliant can help reduce inflammation and restore natural tone.

Herbal Scrubs

Apart from infusing them into essential oils, herbs can also be used as gentle exfoliants. When dried and crushed, plants like rosemary and lavender can be mixed into body scrubs and used as mechanical exfoliants. If your skin is too sensitive and sensitive even for sugar scrubs, you can still use herbal alternatives. Many herbs have antibacterial, antiseptic, and anti-inflammatory effects.

They help soothe irritations, reduce acne and other blemishes, including scars.

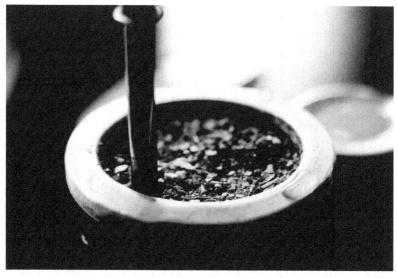

https://unsplash.com/photos/close-up-photography-of-container-ca7YfP8eUj0

Used on your face, herbal scrubs may brighten your complexion by improving its capillary circulation, clearing any skin buildup. They also help combat environmental pollution, which will be visible after the first use. If you are a self-tan enthusiast, you can benefit from herbal scrubs even more. Before applying a self-tanning solution, prep your skin with herbal exfoliation, removing any debris from its surface. This helps even out your skin texture, and you will end up with a more natural-looking tan and an even skin tone. Since the exfoliation also helps absorb moisture, you will need fewer tanning products. Even a smaller amount will provide you with that perfect sun-kissed look, which means applying fewer chemicals to your skin.

Applying plant-based products on your skin also comes with all the medical benefits the particular plants you have used possesses. From simply brightening by cleansing to modifying skin cell structure on a molecular level, if your skin needs healing, herbal scrubs can be an incredibly powerful ally. These scrubs will make your skin radiant and feel smoother than ever before by encouraging collagen production. They are also the perfect way to combat free radicals responsible for premature aging and a number of serious skin conditions. Not only will healthy skin improve your appearance, but it will also better protect you from the environment.

Oatmeal Scrubs

Like herbs, oatmeal can be used as a gentle exfoliator. It's suitable for every skin type and is another common ingredient found in homes. Oatmeal is pretty much already the perfect consistency to become part of your favorite body scrub - and is very effective at removing those layers of dead cells from the top of your skin. When consumed, oats help us maintain our protein and lipid balance and provide us with a number of essential vitamins and minerals. The good news is, using oatmeal as an exfoliant can have the same effect on your skin.

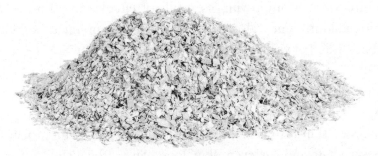

https://unsplash.com/photos/gray-waste-illustration-iYMWwnXC4MU

Vitamin E and zinc are just two of the most powerful anti-inflammatory agents found in nature - and oatmeal has an abundance of them. Due to this, oat scrubs are recommended for people with sensitive skin prone to irritation, itching, and the appearance of painful, red splotches. Even if you have active flare-ups of psoriasis, acne, or eczema, it can be used.

Other crucial ingredients found in oat scrubs are phenols, which form a protective layer on the skin, effectively locking in any moisture under them. Phenols are also responsible for the deep cleansing effect of these scrubs, as they are able to wash away any debris from your skin. This double benefit can be best utilized by combining oatmeal exfoliants with fast-absorbing essential oils, hydrating your skin in just one quick application. Phenols can also improve your appearance by evening out your skin complexion through their antioxidant properties. When applied regularly, oatmeal scrubs help your skin absorb and neutralize harsh environmental factors, including toxic chemicals and UVA rays.

Nut Scrubs

Typically, nut scrubs contain ground nut shells or seeds as exfoliates, which also determine the grit of the scrub. The most commonly used nuts are crushed almonds - which are full of vitamins and minerals necessary to keep your skin healthy and radiant. However, if you have even mild nut allergies, it's best to avoid any type of nuts in your skincare regime. After all, your skin is just as able to absorb its allergy-inducing components as your gastrointestinal system.

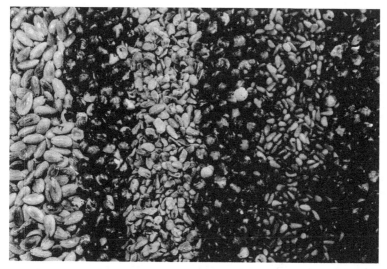

https://unsplash.com/photos/assorted-seed-lot-fZ7-IAReeSo

On the other hand, if you aren't allergic to their components, nut scrubs help maintain skin health and promote healing from existing damage. Regular exfoliation with crushed almonds keeps the skin clean, fades old acne scarring, and reduces the fine lines caused by stress and the natural aging process. Nut exfoliants can be used as a great natural cleanser, especially for improving your complexion by removing any blemishes from your face.

Combined with moisturizing essential oils, nuts also contribute to deep hydration. If your skin is particularly dry, you can use an almond scrub with rich oil and follow up the treatment with an almond-based lotion. This type of reinforced nourishment can be applied to your entire body, including your face. Just make sure to use a suitable face cream after exfoliation. The skin on your face stays hydrated and remains to look fresh due to the antioxidant properties of almonds that improve circulation and prevent impurities.

Turmeric Scrubs

Similar to caffeine, turmeric can also work wonders for your under-eye shadows. While it is often applied in oil form, this spice can also perform as an exfoliant, as long you are using the right type. Make sure you buy the kind that's for external use only, as edible turmeric will stain your skin yellow. The most important benefits of turmeric stem from all the anti-inflammatory and antioxidant properties found in this natural element. This helps combat environmental factors, including the sun's harmful rays - letting you enjoy having smooth, youthful skin. By promoting elastin production, turmeric can ensure your skin remains radiant and wrinkle-free for a long time. In fact, its impact can be so powerful that besides regular moisturizing, exfoliating with turmeric may just turn back time. Turmeric scrubs scrape away dead skin cells very efficiently (which in itself already makes the skin younger) and improve circulation, smoothing out the skin from the first application.

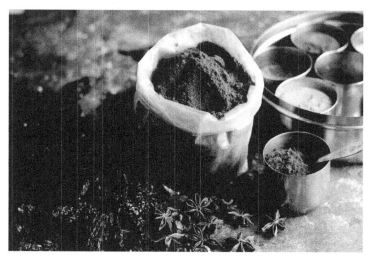

If you are waxing or shaving regularly, you will be happy to know that turmeric can elongate the effects of any hair removal procedure. While the full impacts depend on the hair's texture, the scrub can slow down its growth to a certain extent. Since turmeric also reduces the number of bacteria on your skin, you won't have to worry about razor bumps or ingrown hairs. The same applies to treating severe acne or psoriasis and the inflammation of the affected areas. While both conditions are often treated with steroids and antibiotics, neither medication can provide a long-term solution. On the other hand, naturally, anti-inflammatory agents like turmeric can help solve the issue permanently. It will also help heal the scars caused by past flare-ups and injuries by promoting skin cell growth.

Chapter 3: Oils, Oils, Oils

Now that you know the benefits of exfoliants and their importance as body scrub ingredients, we are going to talk about the other two quintessential elements; carrier oils and essential oils.

Carrier Oils vs. Essential Oils

There are a few differences between carrier oils and essential oils, but the key difference is that carrier oils are safe to use directly on your skin, unlike essential oils. This is because essential oils are highly concentrated and can be too strong to be applied directly to the skin. However, if mixed with carrier oils, essential oils become less concentrated, making them safe to use.

Carrier Oils

The ancient Greeks and Romans were the ones that started using carrier oils for medicines, massages, and baths. Carrier oils are natural oils that are extracted from plants, seeds, and nuts. The secret behind their name, carrier oils, is that they serve as carriers for essential oils to be safely applied to the skin and allow for their spread and absorption as well.

Carrier oils make a great ingredient for homemade body scrubs, especially sugar scrubs. There are different types of carrier oils, so make sure that you choose the type that is right for your skin so it can be more effective. You are probably now wondering which type should you use for your homemade body scrub. Let's take a look at some of the most popular types of carrier oils so you can decide which one you should use.

Sunflower Oil

You have probably heard about the many health benefits of sunflower oil when it comes to preparing healthy and delicious meals. Do you know that it also has many other benefits beyond its use in the kitchen? Sunflower oil can provide your skin with the hydration it needs to stay soft and moisturized. Simply put, when the skin is hydrated, it's able to retain moisture which gives the skin a glow and makes it look healthy. This is why this oil is perfect for people with dry skin. If you have dry skin and add sunflower oil to your body scrub, it will help keep your skin hydrated.

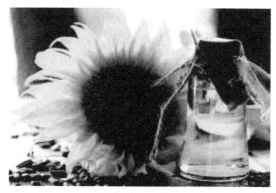

torange.biz, CC BY 4.0 https://creativecommons.org/licenses/by/4.0 via Wikimedia Commons https://commons.wikimedia.org/wiki/File:Sunflower_oil_and_sunflower.jpg

There are so many environmental factors that can harm your skin and cause aging, like UV rays. Sunflower oil works great as an antioxidant since it contains vitamin E, which can protect your skin from pollution and other harmful environmental elements that can damage it and cause rapid aging. Additionally, if you suffer from any kind of skin irritation, then you will really benefit from sunflower's oil soothing properties. It can soothe and moisturize all skin types. If you also have dry or sensitive skin, then you may suffer from occasional temporary redness; this oil can be a great remedy for calming your skin.

Sunflower oil is perfect for all skin types. It keeps dry skin hydrated and moisturized, protects and soothes sensitive skin, balances oils, and moisturizes combination skin. It also balances the oils in oily skin, and unlike other types of oils, sunflower oil doesn't clog pores.

Sesame Oil

As it is clear from the name, Sesame oil is extracted from sesame seeds. Like sunflower oil, sesame oil is also used for cooking, but its benefits don't end there. As we have mentioned before, many elements in the environment can damage your skin, and being exposed to pollution and harmful elements can take a toll on it in the long run. Sesame oil can detoxify your skin, wash away dirt and germs, and rejuvenate your skin to give it a healthy and fresh look. In addition to that, this oil can keep the skin hydrated, moisturized, and smooth. It can also be a solution for cracked heels and moisturizes dry elbows and knees.

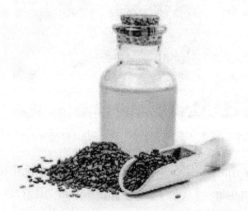

Image by Marco Verch Professional Photographer
https://creativecommons.org/licenses/by/2.0/
https://www.flickr.com/photos/30478819@N08/50813452476/

No one has perfect skin, and many of us suffer from various skin problems. The great thing about sesame oil is that it can help with many of these problems. Suppose you suffer from any skin infection, dead skin, or pimples. In that case, sesame oil can help you get rid of them due to its anti-inflammatory properties. Sesame oil works on all skin types, whether it is dry, sensitive, oily, or a combination.

Olive Oil

You already know the many health benefits olive oils have on your health and hair, but there is more. Olive oil can do wonders to your skin as well. This oil contains different vitamins like vitamins A, D, E, and K, which can all benefit your skin since they can serve as treatments for various skin conditions. Skin requires protection all year long because harsh weather conditions can really take a toll on it. Most skin types suffer during cold weather, especially sensitive ones. The vitamins in olive oil can provide your skin with the protection and nourishment it needs.

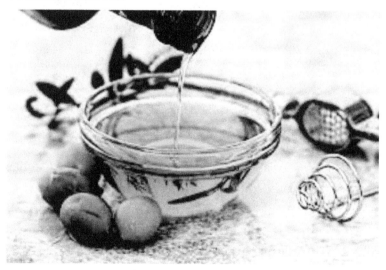

https://pixabay.com/photos/olive-oil-olives-food-oil-natural-968657/

In addition to the vitamins we mentioned above, olive oil contains Omega-3, which provides hydration and slows down the process of aging. It also moisturizes your skin and gives it a healthy glow. Olive oil can be a very beneficial ingredient in your homemade body scrub because if you mix it with sea salt, it can smooth dry skin. That being said, if you have acne-prone or oily skin, then you should stay away from olive oil.

Walnut Oil

You probably know how healthy nuts are (they contain many nutrients!), so it makes sense that oils extracted from them can also provide you with many benefits. There are different types of nuts, but we are going to focus on walnuts and the oil that's extracted from them. Walnut oil can help reduce early signs of aging as it moisturizes the skin, and moisturized and hydrated skin tends to age slower. Additionally, walnuts contain Omega 3, 6, and 9, protecting your skin and giving it a healthy glow.

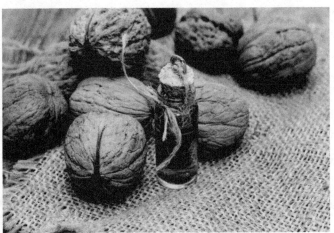

Walnut is a great exfoliating ingredient because it contains vitamin E and antioxidants, which will make your skin look flawless by removing dirt and dead skin. If you have dry skin, then you can really benefit from adding walnut oil to your body scrub. This is because walnut oil is thick, making it perfect for soothing and nourishing dry skin.

Although walnut oil can really benefit your skin, it isn't recommended for everyone. If you are allergic to nuts, then adding walnut oil to your body scrub can be very dangerous. If you aren't sure if you have a nut allergy, you can either opt out of using walnut oil altogether or consult your doctor first. Nut allergies can be very serious, so don't take them lightly.

Now that you know everything about carrier oils and the benefits of some of their most popular oils, we can move on to essential oils.

Essential Oils

Using essential oils isn't something new; people have been using it for centuries, and for good reason! They have many benefits as they can be a treatment for various skin conditions and provide a calming effect. There are different types of essential oils, but we will only cover the ones that can be a great addition to your homemade body scrub.

Orange Oil

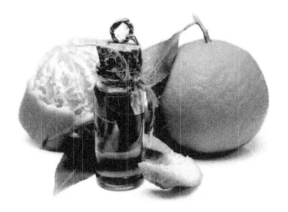

Orange essential oil helps the skin produce collagen, which plays a big role in giving you a youthful look and reducing the signs of aging. In addition to that, orange oil removes any toxins from your skin which evens its tone and makes it look clean and fresh. This oil can also add a fruity scent to your body scrub, which will help you smell nice all day. You can use sweet orange oil on all types of skin, but you should be careful with bitter orange oil. Essential oils extracted from bitter oranges can cause a severe reaction to your skin if you are exposed to the sun. Therefore, they are better used at night.

Neroli Oil

Neroli oil comes from the flowers of bitter orange trees. This oil can bring dull skin back to life and help reduce many skin issues like wrinkles, scars, and stretch marks. Adding neroli to your homemade body scrub won't only benefit your skin but your body as well. Most, if not all, women know how painful PMS can be, and they are always looking for something to reduce the pain. When you add neroli oil to your body scrub and rub your body with it, it can relieve the pain. It can help people who are suffering from colon problems as well. Neroli oil is perfect for people with oily skin because it soothes and moisturizes.

Peppermint Oil

Peppermint oil contains many healthy minerals like calcium, potassium, magnesium, iron, and Omega-3. These minerals can benefit your skin and give you a youthful look. In addition to that, it can also soothe your skin and make you feel refreshed. As you probably know, just the smell of peppermint can make you feel refreshed, so imagine how it will make you feel when it's applied to your skin. Peppermint oil can also be very beneficial to people who are suffering from acne since it limits oil production in the skin.

That being said, you should be careful when using peppermint oil. Yes, it has many benefits, but too much of it can harm your skin. Only opt for a few drops on your homemade scrub, or your skin may be irritated. Additionally, you may be allergic to peppermint oil and don't even know it, so it is recommended to test it first.

Chamomile Oil

Chamomile has always been known for its soothing effects, which is why people drink chamomile tea when they need to calm down. Oil extracted from this plant can soothe skin irritation, itches, and sunburn. It can also be very beneficial to dry skin, especially during the cold weather when your skin needs extra hydration. This oil also promotes relaxation as it can reduce stress and elevate your mood, which is why many pregnant women use it to help them relax. Adding chamomile oil to your buddy scrub and showering with it before bed can help you relax, which will make you sleep better at night.

Rose Oil

What sets rose oil apart from the other types of oil we have mentioned here is that it is more expensive. If you have bought a bouquet of flowers recently, then you know that roses don't come cheap. The price may be worth it since the oil will provide more than a floral scent to your homemade scrub. Rose oil can help hydrate and moisturize your skin, which can slow down the aging process, make you look youthful, and give you glowing skin. Additionally, this oil can improve your mood as a result of its floral smell. It also reduces stress and makes you feel relaxed. You can use this oil on all skin types, but people with dry and mature skin will benefit from it the most.

Frankincense

Frankincense oil is extracted from Boswellia trees in India. This oil has many health benefits to your body and skin. Frankincense oil can reduce the signs of aging on your skin, along with scars and acne. It can also help lift your spirits, which is why so many people prefer to use it during the winter because gloomy weather can negatively impact their mood. Although it can benefit all types of skin, people with mature skin reap its benefits the most since it soothes and moisturizes the skin. It is important to note that you should only use a few drops of this oil because if you overdo it, it can be toxic.

Now that you know about different types of carriers and essential oils, you can easily pick the right ones for your skin. If you are pregnant, you should know that there are essential oils that you should steer clear of since they may do more harm than good.

Avoid These Essential Oils If You Are Pregnant

Rosemary Oil

Rosemary oil can cause problems for pregnant women if used in high doses.

Birch Oil

Birch oil contains methyl salicylate, which pregnant women should steer clear of.

Wintergreen Oil

Like Birch oil, wintergreen oil contains methyl salicylate, which is why you should avoid it if you are pregnant.

Cinnamon Oil

Cinnamon oil can be dangerous for the mother and the baby and can cause serious complications.

Generally, it is better to avoid all essential oils while pregnant because they may negatively affect the baby or cause early contractions. If you must use them, then ask your doctor first, but it is better to be safe than sorry and avoid using them completely until another time.

Chapter 4: Coffee Body Scrubs

Coffee can do much more than wake you in the morning and provide your daily dose of productive boost. This magical ingredient contains a plethora of useful skin benefits that can help improve its texture and health. Due to its versatility, coffee can be blended with several other skincare ingredients to make a super-effective body scrub recipe. In this chapter, we will take a look at some effective coffee body scrub recipes for you to choose from based on your preferences and skin goals. Before that, let's dive into several benefits of using coffee.

Benefits of Coffee in Body Scrubs

Despite being an effective cellulite-fighter, coffee is one of the most underrated skincare ingredients in body scrub recipes. It offers the following skin benefits.

1. Rich in Antioxidants

Coffee grounds are rich in antioxidants, which can be used to fight free radicals and premature aging, thereby giving the skin an even tone and a youthful look. Failing to detoxify your skin can result in breakage of collagen, which can cause rapid aging. This, in turn, can result in wrinkly and saggy skin at an early age. Coffee can also reduce the effects of harmful UV rays and pollution. Additionally, it helps dehydrate fat cells by acting on the fast-breaking enzymes.

2. Increases Blood Circulation and Promotes Even Complexion

Caffeine is also known to enhance blood circulation to promote an even complexion. Using any kind of coffee scrub for a few months can help you achieve smooth and moisturized skin for a long time. If you suffer from hyperpigmentation, exfoliating your body with a coffee scrub can also reduce dark spots and help you achieve permanent results. With every exfoliation session, you are helping your skin breathe and further allowing the product to sink in due to the elimination of dead skin cells. As the fresh skin cells appear on top, your skin automatically looks even-toned and brighter. Caffeine encourages microcirculation, which keeps blood vessels tight and treats pigmentation and discoloration.

3. Acts as a Great Exfoliator

The skin readily absorbs the good properties of coffee grounds, which enhances the exfoliation process and removes dead skin cells with ease. Coffee's sand-like texture also rejuvenates the skin and helps with even exfoliation. Removing dead cells can help improve your skin's texture; your skin will feel smoother and softer. If used regularly, coffee is also known to reduce the effects of keratosis pilaris, a common skin issue causing tiny bumps, scars, and rough patches. This usually occurs at the back of the arms and on the hips.

4. Treats Inflammation

Coffee contains two important anti-inflammatory components, which are hydrocinnamic acid and polyphenols. Any kind of inflammation, red scars, or breakouts can be treated using a topical application of coffee. It specifically treats inflamed body parts caused by extreme sun exposure and sun damage. Essentially, coffee can also be used to treat puffiness and reduce undereye bags, which make you look sleepy and tired. The caffeine content in coffee tightens or constricts your blood vessels, which reduces puffiness. This is also why caffeine is known as a vasoconstrictor, which can also help brighten your skin. You can use fine ground coffee to scrub your face. However, massage gently under your eyes to avoid your skin from peeling. When paired with other ingredients like chamomile and green tea, coffee scrubs can act as an effective stimulant to treat inflammation.

5. Reduces Stretch Marks and Fights Cellulite

One of the most important benefits of using coffee in body scrubs is the reduction of cellulite and stretch marks. Any kind of fine lines, freckles, marks, and sunspots can be treated topically by applying coffee. It may take some time for the spots to disappear, but the results are long-lasting and permanent. The stimulating effect of caffeine helps your fat cells shrink in size, which reduces the white spots and uneven texture caused by cellulite.

Now that you are aware of various skin benefits promoted by coffee, you can use this versatile ingredient as a skincare stimulant and include it in your daily routine.

Coffee Body Scrub Recipes

You can make a lot of varieties of coffee scrubs with ingredients that are readily available in your pantry. These DIY recipes are easy to make, take just a few minutes to prepare, and can be stored in air-tight containers for up to two to three months (the shelf life can vary according to the type of ingredients used).

Coffee, Sugar, and Coconut Scrub

This coffee body scrub recipe reduces cellulite and tightens the skin. Coconut oil is also another fantastic skincare ingredient due to its moisturizing properties and anti-aging boosters. Sugar acts as a natural exfoliator and squeezes out dead skin cells, thereby giving you a smooth and even skin texture. You can also add a few drops of vanilla extract to enhance the mixture's scent. Cinnamon is another optional ingredient that stimulates blood circulation and improves the mixture's aroma.

Ingredients

- Ground coffee- 1 cup or approximately 120 grams
- Brown sugar- ½ cup or approximately 65 grams
- Melted organic coconut oil (cold-pressed) - ½ cup or 120 ml
- Vanilla extract- 1 tsp or 5 ml
- Ground cinnamon- 1 tsp or 5 grams

Where to Find the Ingredients

You can find the main ingredients at any convenience store near you. For all recipes, use organic coffee to get the best results. Use cold-pressed virgin coconut oil for this recipe. It is a bit more expensive than regular coconut oil, but the amazing results make it worthwhile. Instead of white sugar, get brown cane sugar from your local grocery store for better results.

Directions

1. Add ground coffee and sugar to a bowl and mix thoroughly. If you use huge coffee grounds, you may have to whisk them together using a blender or a whisk attachment.

2. Keep beating the mixture until the coffee breaks evenly and all ingredients are blended well. The mixture should get fluffy, soft, and slightly grainy.

3. Add vanilla extract and coconut oil. Mix well until the mixture turns into a paste. If needed, add more coconut oil to make a semi-solid paste such that it is easy to spread on your body.

4. You can use it directly under the shower or store it in an air-tight container to be used for up to 2 months.

Coconut oil can be extremely sticky and greasy, so you must wash your body with soap after exfoliating it with this scrub. If you have oily skin, do not use coconut oil as it can cause breakouts and acne. Replace it with almond oil or a small amount of cold-pressed olive oil.

Coffee and Vitamin E Scrub

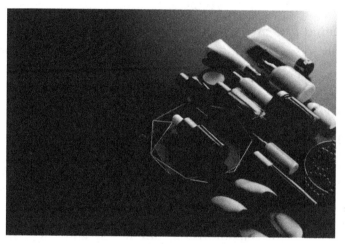

https://unsplash.com/photos/a-table-topped-with-lots-of-different-types-of-cosmetics-ILhf4VsPn_w

Skin experts suggest applying the combination of coffee and Vitamin E as it is rich in antioxidants and fights free radicals. Vitamin E, in particular, can nourish your skin when applied topically. This ingredient's anti-aging properties also make it a great addition to your coffee scrub. It also moisturizes your skin and prevents itching. Almond oil treats scars and provides an even complexion. If used properly and regularly, it can also reverse the effects of sun damage. We are also adding brown sugar and orange essential oil to this recipe for additional skin benefits.

Ingredients

- Ground coffee- 1 cup or approximately 120 grams

- Vitamin E oil- ½ tsp or 2.5 ml

- Almond oil- ½ tsp or 2.5 ml

- Brown sugar- ½ cup or approximately 65 grams

- Orange or any other essential oil of your choice- 10 to 15 drops

Where to Find the Ingredients

Vitamin E is available in the form of oil and can be applied topically to your skin. Ensure that the brand and type of oil you buy is authentic, and beware of fake suppliers. You can easily find high-quality Vitamin E oil and almond oil at your nearest pharmacy or a convenience store—order orange essential oil on an online store or a local beauty shop.

Directions

1. Add ground coffee and sugar to a bowl and mix thoroughly using a hand blender or a whisker.

2. Add Vitamin E oil, almond oil, and a few drops of orange essential oil. Mix well until you achieve your desired texture.

3. Store it in an air-tight container to be used for up to 1 or 2 months.

You can increase the amount of almond oil to make the paste smoother and thinner. To enhance its aroma, add a few more drops of your favorite essential oil.

Coffee and Shea Butter Scrub

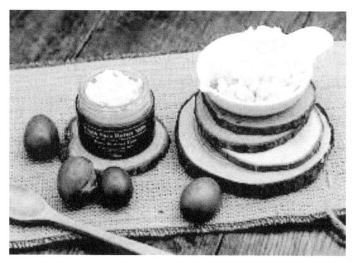

Hopkinsuniv, CC BY-SA 3.0 https://creativecommons.org/licenses/by-sa/3.0 via Wikimedia Commons https://commons.wikimedia.org/wiki/File:Sheabutter-virginsheabutter.jpg

Another effective skincare ingredient, shea butter, is extracted from shea tree kernels and has several skincare benefits. Due to its hydrating and moisturizing properties, it is excessively used in face creams and body moisturizers. It is abundant in several useful fatty acids, like stearic, oleic, linoleic, and palmitic acids. It also reduces harmful effects caused by sun damage, pollutants, and excessive sun exposure. Since shea butter is also rich in anti-inflammatory properties, the combination of coffee and shea butter is extremely useful to treat skin inflammation and puffiness. Shea butter also treats anti-aging issues and breakouts.

Ingredients

- Ground coffee- 1 cup or approximately 120 grams
- Raw shea butter- 2 tbsp or approximately 30 grams
- Almond oil- ½ tsp or 2.5 ml
- Ground cinnamon- 1 tsp or 5 grams

How and Where to Find the Ingredients

Since you already know the right way to buy ground coffee and almond oil for your coffee scrub, let's talk about the new ingredient, shea butter. It is categorized into two types: East African and West African. Even though both types of shea butter are useful to treat and moisturize your skin, you can pick one based on specific skin requirements and goals. West African shea butter is abundant in Vitamin A and can be used to treat wrinkles, blemishes, and scars. On the other hand, East African shea butter is more suitable for wounds, dry skin, and sensitive skin. Buy shea butter in a raw and unrefined form for best results as it is free of preservatives and chemicals. You can find it at a local beauty or organic store. Unrefined shea butter is also readily available on Amazon.

Directions

1. Put shea butter in a microwavable container and melt it for 30 seconds.

2. Add almond oil to it and mix properly. Let the mixture sit for a while until the oil gets slightly soft and firm. This will also keep the coffee grounds from settling at the bottom.

3. Add coffee grounds and cinnamon powder to the mixture and mix properly. You can also add a pinch of salt to enhance its texture.

Suppose you suffer from dry skin throughout the year. In that case, this coffee scrub using shea butter as a special ingredient will keep your body moisturized and soft. Since you are using raw shea butter in this recipe, it may lack fragrance. However, the addition of almond oil and cinnamon will provide a light and fresh fragrance to your scrub. If you are allergic to tree nuts, avoid using shea butter. If used excessively, it can also clog pores. However, almond oil, being non-comedogenic, can treat clogged pores. Its high Vitamin E content is also useful to treat skin issues and make it softer.

Coffee and Pumpkin Spice Essential Oils Scrub

Certain types of essential oils improve skin texture, treat hyperpigmentation, and provide an even complexion. Nutmeg and clove bud oils are antibacterial and anti-inflammatory in nature. They make great additions to any skincare product. Ginger essential oil is also rich in antioxidants and can help flush out harmful toxins while treating redness and inflammation. It also helps reduce fine lines and wrinkles. Rich in vitamins and fatty acids, shea nut oil can help moisturize your skin and reduce flakiness. Cassia oil is another useful essential oil for your skin, which treats sores, wounds, and acne.

Ingredients

- Ground coffee- 1 cup or approximately 120 grams
- Brown sugar- ½ cup or approximately 65 grams
- Ginger Essential Oil- 2 drops
- Clove Bud Essential Oil- 4 drops
- Nutmeg Essential Oil- 4 drops
- Shea Nut Oil- 2 tbsp or approximately 30 ml
- Cassia Bark Essential Oil- 4 drops

Where to Find the Ingredients

All essential oils can be found in a local beauty store or an online store.

Directions

1. Add ground coffee and sugar to a bowl and mix thoroughly using a hand blender or a whisker.

2. Add a few drops of all essential oils and mix well until you achieve your desired texture.

3. Store it in an air-tight container to be used for up to one or two months.

Before adding the essential oils to the mixture, do a patch test to check if you are allergic to any ingredient. Since some types of essential oil can cause skin redness and irritation, check all potential ingredients before you add them to your scrub recipe by doing a patch test.

Coffee and Green Tea Scrub

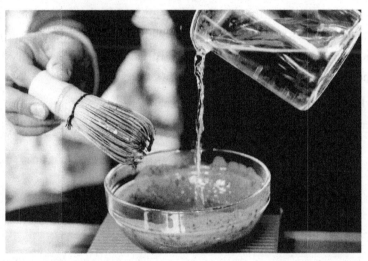

https://unsplash.com/photos/person-pouring-water-into-green-sauce-f3uWanPu_rU

Green tea is known for its antioxidant properties, which is why it is excessively used in the fitness and skincare world. It can help remove toxins from the skin and treat pigmentation. This is also why green tea extract is a popular ingredient in face creams today. Add Epsom salt to the mixture if you constantly suffer from sore muscles and internal inflammation. Jojoba oil hydrates your skin without making it oily.

Ingredients

- Ground coffee- 1 cup or approximately 120 grams
- Baking soda- 2 tsp or approximately 8 grams
- Epsom salt- 3 tsp or approximately 13 grams

- Jojoba oil- 4 drops

- Green tea- 1 bag

Where to Find the Ingredients

Typically, Epsom salt can be found in pharmacies. When buying it, make sure that the brand and product are certified and tested by the relevant organization in your region. Pick organic green tea bags from your local grocery or organic store. Jojoba oil can be bought from an online beauty store or through Amazon.

Directions

1. Boil one cup of water and place the green tea bag in it. Let it steep for a few minutes.

2. Brew the mixture and keep it aside. Mix baking soda, Epsom salt, and ground coffee in a separate bowl.

3. Add the brewed tea and a few drops of Jojoba oil. Mix well and store it in a container.

You can adjust the quantity of any ingredient for additional skin benefits or to achieve your desired texture. Use this mixture on your feet to fight foot odor.

Bonus Recipe: 3-Ingredient Easy Coffee Scrub

To make a simple coffee scrub within a few minutes, mix 1 cup of fine coffee with 3 tbsp (around 40 grams) of aloe vera and 1 tsp (around 5 ml) of rose water. Mix well to form a smooth paste and use it as a scrub before showering. You can also add two drops of juniper seed oil for its antiseptic properties.

How to Use This Coffee Body Scrub

Ideally, body scrubs should be used once or twice a week. Depending on your needs and preferences, you can use one of these body scrub recipes to exfoliate your skin once a week. Apply it once a week if you simply want to achieve smoother skin. However, if you are treating your skin for cellulite reduction or hyperpigmentation, use one of these recipes at least twice or three times a week. Typically, 1-2 tbsp of any coffee body scrub mixture is enough to exfoliate your entire body. Wet your skin before applying the scrub. Spread the mixture onto your arms and legs and gently massage in a circular motion for a few minutes. This will help remove all dead and dry skin and open all pores. Do not rub it harshly or aggressively.

You must use one of these coffee scrubs throughout the year and not just in summer. Even though the rough texture of the coffee scrub can cause flaky skin during winter, do not stop using it. Apply extra moisturizer after you have finished exfoliating and scrubbing. You should specifically use a coffee scrub during winter to get rid of flaky and dry skin. During summer, as soon as you step inside after spending a hot day outdoors, use a coffee scrub before showering to remove excess sunscreen and sweat.

Use a paper towel to remove as many coffee granules as you can. Use warm water to rinse off the remaining scrub mixture and apply soap to remove the oiliness from coconut oil, essential oils, and other additional ingredients. Since coffee grounds can clog your drain, place a filter on top to catch the particles. Store all scrub mixtures in an air-tight container and place them in a cold and dry spot. Use them within two months. To extend the shelf-life, you may have to add some kind of preservatives. However, it is recommended to use them in their freshest and most natural form.

Warnings and Precautions

Since coffee grounds can be abrasive, you must apply a small amount on every body part when scrubbing. Do not scrub excessively, as it can damage or peel the skin. Note that exfoliating and scrubbing your skin does not guarantee instant results. You must exfoliate your skin using this coffee scrub every week for a few months to notice improved blood circulation and reduction in spots, acne, stretch marks, and cellulite. Most importantly, use a moisturizer once you have finished scrubbing your body for the pores to absorb moisture. Failing to use a moisturizer can make your skin dry and rough over time.

Do not use any coffee scrub on your face as it is abrasive on sensitive skin. If you still want to use a coffee face scrub, replace coffee particles or grounds with fine ground coffee. Since coarse grounds can damage skin over time, stick to fine grounds to make your body scrub as well.

Add one of these coffee scrubs to your skincare routine, especially if your skin goal is fighting cellulite and reducing stretch marks. Coffee's texture can help you achieve glowing skin with a radiant appearance. If you love the smell of coffee, this scrub is definitely for you. Don't just drink your daily cup of Joe - use it in your skincare routine as well. If used wisely, coffee scrubs can also be applied to your face and scalp to achieve similar results. Regular usage of a coffee scrub will result in smoother, firmer, and brighter skin.

Chapter 5: Oatmeal Body Scrubs

Oatmeal is rich in vitamins and minerals and is beneficial for reducing inflammation and oxidative stress. Apart from being one of the healthiest breakfast options, oats have been used for skincare for thousands of years in various forms. Ancient Egyptians took healing oat baths to cure skin conditions and mixed oats into other skincare products, including body scrubs. This chapter contains several oatmeal scrub recipes suitable for different uses. Before you dive into making and trying out your own oatmeal scrubs, you will need to understand how they can benefit your skin.

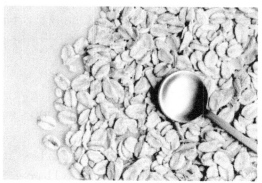

https://unsplash.com/photos/brown-rice-on-white-textile-caPcNn41FnY

Benefits of Oatmeal Body Scrubs

Since it's very gentle on the skin, oatmeal can be used for all skin types. Regular exfoliation with oatmeal scrubs will result in the following benefits.

Cleansing and Exfoliation

Oatmeal gives body scrubs a finer grit, allowing them to be gentler on the skin. Whether you have oily, dry, sensitive, or blemish-prone skin, oatmeal can help in keeping it polished and smooth. Oats could be the perfect solution if you are looking for a natural ingredient that will exfoliate your skin without stripping it of all the moisture – as many store-bought products do. Furthermore, oatmeal scrubs are suitable for the face and body - although their use may depend on the other ingredients as well. Thanks to the saponin content in the oats, these scrubs are super easy to lather, making their application for cleansing a breeze.

Irritation and Blemish Relief

Oatmeal scrubs are found most beneficial by those who have sensitive skin that's prone to irritations and blemishes. Oats contain avenanthramides - compounds with antiseptic properties. They help reduce the number of bacteria on your skin, preventing acne and other blemishes. In case you already have an existing skin condition that causes irritation or inflammation, these same amazing components will reduce it, relieving your symptoms after just a couple of uses. Oatmeal is famous for its moisture absorbing capacity, which you can also use for stripping the excess oils from your skin.

Anti-Aging Effects

A thick layer of dead cell buildup on the surface of your skin can make you look aged. Oats can remove all those layers and reveal smooth skin free of age spots, dry patches, and fine lines that often make you appear much older. Homemade oatmeal scrubs are typically made of very few organic ingredients, which make them perfect for frequent use. It allows you to turn back time and revitalize your skin very quickly. Not only can oatmeal scrubs combat signs of natural aging, but they also revive skin that's been damaged by excess sunbathing.

Moisturizing

Oats can leave your skin looking plump and hydrated despite their high moisture absorbing capacity. This is because they contain high amounts of essential lipids. When reaching your skin, they can integrate into it, providing an instant moisturizing effect. While applying a skin-appropriate lotion is recommended after scrubbing, oatmeal scrubs alone can work wonders on restoring a healthy skin tone. They will also help maintain it as stripping away layers of dead cells allows your skin to retain significantly more moisture from lotions and creams. Even if you have extremely dry skin and are prone to atopic eczema, or psoriasis, the lipids from the oatmeal will keep it hydrated.

Oatmeal Scrubs

Oats are one of the most budget-friendly ingredients for a homemade exfoliant – and they are also the most *versatile ones*. Here are some easy face and body scrub recipes using oats or oatmeal.

Honey Lavender Cleanser

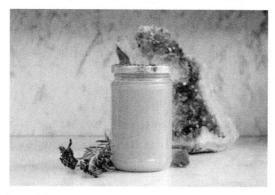

https://unsplash.com/photos/a-jar-of-orange-juice-next-to-a-purple-flower-kMa9ILOsljk

Using lavender cleansers is great to soothe sensitive skin at any time of the year. Whether you have suffered a skin burn, have atopic eczema, or just very dry skin in the winter, lavender essential oils can be the perfect solution. The scent of lavender is one of those fragrances that make you feel better just from smelling it - imagine putting it on your skin in a concentrated form. Combined with oatmeal and honey, this essential oil makes a gentle yet moisturizing cleanser no one can resist. Powdered milk is the perfect way to add protein and other nutrients to your skin and help it heal.

Ingredients

- Powdered milk - 1 tbsp or approximately 8 grams
- Oatmeal - 1 tbsp or 9.5 grams
- Honey - 1 tbsp or 15 ml
- Lavender essential oil - 2 drops or 0.1 ml
- Water - 2 tbsp or 30 ml

Where to Find the Ingredients

You will find oatmeal, powdered milk, and honey in any convenience store. In case you want to substitute powdered milk for plant-based milk powders, you will get these in better-supplied supermarkets or health food stores. Pure lavender essential oil is typically sold in beauty supply stores, where you can make sure it has truly organic origins.

Directions

- First, place the dry ingredients (raw oatmeal and powdered milk) in a large bowl, and mix them until well combined.

- Pour in the water, and mix again to dissolve the powdered milk. When the milk begins to bubble, and you can clearly smell it, mix in the honey as well.

- Once your mixture reaches a paste-like consistency, mix in 1-2 drops of lavender essential oils. It's a very fragrant oil, so you may find that even one drop will be enough.

- Use the mixture right away or within two days. If you have prepared it ahead, keep it refrigerated until finished. Otherwise, the milk will get spoiled.

Oatmeal Treatment with Grapefruit

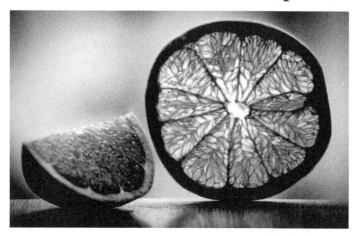

https://unsplash.com/photos/a-grapefruit-cut-in-half-on-a-table-6HsStlFXK-k

If you have oily, acne-prone skin, you will need this scrub in your beauty regimen. It will be particularly beneficial during hot summer days when you still need to moisturize - but you need a refreshing product to do so. Grapefruit can help you do that, and it will also provide you with plenty of vitamins. Combined with brown sugar, the acidity of the grapefruit can strip the skin of excess oils, which is necessary to prevent blemishes. The recipe also uses ready-made oatmeal, so you won't have to worry about grinding it. Plus, the formula has one huge advantage: it's completely edible.

Ingredients

- Oatmeal - 1 cup or 80 grams

- Brown sugar - 1 tbsp or approximately 12 grams

- Grapefruit juice - 1-2 tbsp or

- Water - as needed

Where to Find the Ingredients

There's a good chance you may already have oatmeal and brown sugar at home. If you don't, rest assured that you will be able to find them in any convenience store. Typically, the same is true for grapefruits, which should naturally be organic and pesticide-free. While you can buy ready-made grapefruit juice as well, there is nothing better than freshly squeezed fruit juice. It contains a lot more vitamins and antioxidants and is free of any preservatives.

Directions

1. Pour the oatmeal into a large bowl and mix it with the brown sugar until well combined. You will know it's evenly mixed when you can no longer find lumps of sugar.

2. Once the dry ingredient is mixed, you can squeeze in the grapefruit juice and start adding in water. Stop after about one tablespoon, and mix it well.

3. Keep adding water until you get a homogenous structure. If you want to use it on your body, you will need a more spreadable formula. For your face, you may keep it slightly thicker.

4. Once you are satisfied with the consistency, the treatment will be ready to use for your face or your body. Store it in a moderately cool place until used or for a couple of days.

Almond Oat Scrub

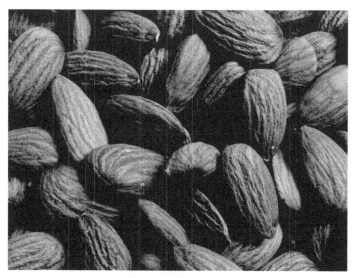

https://unsplash.com/photos/brown-and-green-oval-leaves-wdJaZR4PCeg

Like most oatmeal scrubs, this one is also easy to prepare. It uses almond oil to make your skin silky and perfectly moisturized, while the milk adds essential proteins that promote regeneration. This formula is perfect for healing scars, burns and even works on stretch marks. Another great thing about this recipe is that if you are sensitive to any of its components, you can easily swap them for safer ones. For example, if you have nut allergies, you can always substitute almond oil with avocado oil. You can also use any other type of milk. Oat milk can be a great alternative as it's plant-based, has similar protein content as regular milk, and is usually safe to use for everyone.

Ingredients

- Oats - 1/2 cup or 45 grams
- Almond oil - 1/4 cup or 60ml
- Milk - 1/4 cup or 60ml
- Water - as needed
- Honey - 1 tsp or 5ml

Where to Find the Ingredients

You can acquire most of the ingredients from the nearest convenience store. While some of them also offer almond oil, you may find a better-quality oil in a local beauty supply store. Make sure you buy an organic almond oil that's safe to use on the skin. If you decide to swap it for avocado or olive oil, you may find those in the supermarket as well.

Directions

1. Put the oats in a blender or food processor and grind them until they reach a fine grit. This will allow for a smoother application, which this formula requires. For the same reason, it's best to mix the entire scrub in the blender as well.

2. When you are satisfied with the grit, pour in the honey and add the almond oil and milk in small increments. Don't add more than a teaspoon of liquid at a time so that the blender can incorporate it properly.

3. The final consistency of the mixture should be easily spreadable. If you run out of oil and milk before it reaches this state, you can add water until you are satisfied with the consistency.

4. Once you have reached the desired consistency, you can use the scrub right away. You can use it on your entire body and face, including your under-eye area.

5. If there is any left, make sure you keep it refrigerated until finished. Due to its milk content, the scrub is only safe to use within two days.

Coconut Oatmeal Scrub

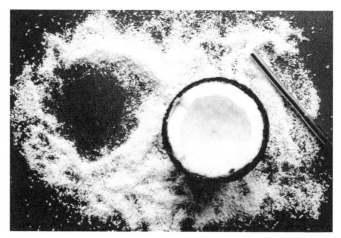

https://unsplash.com/photos/white-and-brown-round-ornament-H8S3Gx_SZoI

Coconut oil is not only helpful in preparing healthy meals, but it can leave your skin incredibly smooth and smelling fantastic. Combined with oats, this is simple oil that you can whip up any time your skin needs pampering, and it makes a very inexpensive scrub. Even if it's just your hands and feet that need scrubbing, you can make them softer than ever in no time at all. The formula contains no fragrance, which means it is suitable for all skin types. If you have very sensitive skin that is easily irritated by any fragrances, this formula will be very soothing. It's also a great exfoliant to use during pregnancy and breastfeeding.

Ingredients

- Oats - 1 1/2 cup or 135 grams
- Coconut oil - 1/2 cup or 118 ml
- Brown sugar - 1 tsp or approximately 12 grams
- Honey - 1 tsp or 5ml

Where to Find the Ingredients

If you don't already have them in your pantry, you can find all the ingredients in any well-supplied convenience store. Ensure all the products you buy for this recipe are organic, particularly if you have sensitive skin or are pregnant. If you fall into these categories, it's best to use colloidal oatmeal that's already milled into a fine grit so that it will be even more delicate on your skin.

Directions

1. Put the oats in a blender or food processor and blend them until you are satisfied with their texture. The particles should be no larger than sugar granules, but if you can grind them smaller, that's even better. You can skip this step and move directly to the next one when using colloidal oatmeal.

2. Heat the coconut oil in a microwave for about 45 seconds or until it's liquefied.

3. Pour the ground oats into a large bowl, add sugar, and mix it until well combined. The sugar should be evenly coated with the finer particles of the oatmeal.

4. Add the honey, then slowly start adding the coconut oil as well. You mustn't add all the liquid at once, as doing so will make it harder to mix.

5. When you have added the last of the coconut oil, you should have a smooth mixture, ready to use after a shower or bath. You can use it on your face, but avoid the area around your eyes.

6. You can store any leftovers in a moderately cold environment for 2-3 months.

Cinnamon Oatmeal Scrub with Vanilla Extract

If you have skin that's on the drier side, you will love this recipe, especially during the winter months. Although it's made from a combination of several different exfoliants and healthy fats, it may be suitable for other skin types. The oats and the sugar will provide your delicate skin with gentle cleansing and antioxidants, while the oils will make sure your skin stays soft and moisturized. What makes this scrub even more perfect for winter use are the spices that will make you think of cinnamon cookie dough. If you can restrain yourself from tasting it, feel free to try it on your skin.

Ingredients

- White sugar - 3/4 cup or 150 grams

- Oats -3/4 cup or 117 grams

- Brown sugar - ¾ cup or 160 grams

- Coconut oil - 1/2 cup or approximately 120 ml

- Olive oil - 1/4 cup

- Vanilla extract - 1 tsp or 5ml

- Cinnamon - 1/2 tsp or approximately 2.8 grams

Where to Find the Ingredients

Most of the ingredients can be found in your local supermarket. Since the recipe also uses sugar, the grit will already be a little harsher, so you can use regular raw oats for this recipe. It's recommended to use virgin olive oil and cold-pressed coconut oil as these are even richer in essential fats. Use only organic, liquid vanilla extract and organic cinnamon to make your skin smell delicious for hours afterward.

Directions

1. Place the oats in a blender or food processor and blend them until you get particles no larger than sugar granules. The bigger the particles are, the harsher the exfoliation will be.

2. Put the coconut oil in the microwave for about 45 seconds or until it becomes completely liquid. Alternatively, you can melt it in a pan, but the process will be much slower.

3. While the coconut oil is heating up, combine the oats with the sugars and the cinnamon in a large bowl, followed by the olive oil and the vanilla extract.

4. Pour the coconut oil onto the mixture while it's hot, and make sure you mix it as quickly as possible. You mustn't delay this step because cooling down will cause the coconut oil to solidify again.

5. You can use the scrub immediately after showering and store the leftovers in a glass container. Kept in a moderately cold place (not in the fridge), it has a shelf-life of up to 3 months.

How to Use Oatmeal Scrubs

Keep in mind that depending on the other ingredients used in them, only some of these oatmeal scrubs may be suitable for your body and face, whereas some formulas are to be applied to your body only. For further information, please check the individual recipes. Most oatmeal scrubs can be used up to twice a week, making them easy to incorporate into your regular beauty routine. Exfoliating with oats once a week will suffice if you have normal skin. People suffering from conditions like psoriasis, eczema, or severe acne may benefit from more frequent use, especially during colder months. If you have particularly oily skin, you can apply a suitable oatmeal scrub 1-2 times a week - depending on the current condition of your skin. Since heat tends to aggravate sebum production, you may need to use the products more frequently during the summer. Regardless of your skin type, it's recommended to use oatmeal scrubs at least once a week. This will help maintain a polished and youthful look for years to come.

For the best results, apply oatmeal scrubs after a shower or a bath while your skin is still damp. Take a nice dollop and massage it gently into your skin. If you have used a finer grit and your skin isn't too sensitive, you can use an exfoliating mitt to ensure the formula cleanses all your pores. If your skin is irritated, itching, or painful to touch, tap the formula onto it gently using your fingertips. Since oatmeal does not dissolve completely, as salt or sugar scrubs would, it will be necessary to wait five minutes after application. During this time, the oats will strip away all the debris from your skin, allowing your skin to absorb the essential oils. After this, you can wash away the scrub with lukewarm water. Soak it a little bit before beginning to wipe it down with your hands to help remove all the particles.

Disclaimers

Oatmeal is considered one of the healthiest and safest items you can put on your skin. Compared to sugar or salt scrubs, oats as exfoliants carry far fewer side effects. However, due to the other ingredients contained in oatmeal scrubs, some of these recipes may require you to take certain precautions. Needless to say, if you are sensitive to any of the components and it cannot be substituted for another one, that particular product is not safe for you to use. You should avoid using essential oils on your body while pregnant and breastfeeding, as they may cause hormonal imbalance. Opt for a recipe with vanilla or similar natural extract if you want your scrub to be fragrant.

When making DIY oatmeal face and body scrubs, it's recommended to use *colloidal* oatmeal. This is made from oats that are ground to a specific grit that's suitable for topical application. While you can use regular oatmeal or even blend raw oats on your own, this may not give you the desired results. A blender intended for home use will only grind the oats to a medium grit that's only applicable on certain skin types. It's definitely not good to use it on irritated skin, as it will hurt your skin and further aggravate your condition. On the other hand, colloidal oatmeal will allow you to create a fine grit that you can safely use on all skin types and conditions. If, despite this, you notice that your symptoms are getting worse, stop using the body scrub and consult your dermatologist for possible relief.

Chapter 6: Salt Body Scrubs

Combined with the perfect carrier and essential oils, salts can be the perfect solution for polishing your skin. The most common types of salt used in body scrubs are Mediterranean, Himalayan, Dead Sea, and Hawaiian salts. Different salts have different beneficial properties, which you can explore when making your own scrubs. Their mineral content includes varying amounts of magnesium, calcium, iron, potassium, and copper. In this chapter, you will find a few simple, organic recipes that highlight all of the amazing benefits salt body scrubs can provide your body with. Despite their low preparation costs, these exfoliators can help facilitate the pampering you need. You will also be given an overview of the advantages and possible disadvantages of using salt body scrubs for exfoliation.

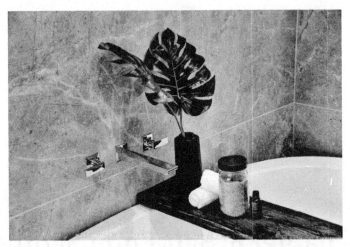

https://unsplash.com/photos/green-plant-on-brown-wooden-table-lWqmnx1DUSk

Benefits of Salt Body Scrubs

There are several reasons why salts are often praised by those who use them frequently. When used in body scrubs, salts can provide an ultimate spa-like experience. Here are some of the benefits you can take advantage of in the comfort of your home.

Mechanical Exfoliation

Due to their texture, most salts are perfect for harsh mechanical exfoliation. During this process, they remove layers of dead cells from the skin's surface, revealing the new layers underneath. Unlike the dead layers, which often appear flaky, hard, dry, and often discolored, the new skin has an even tone as it is smooth to touch. The longer you wait between two exfoliation treatments, the more layers will be removed, and the results will be even more astonishing. However, thicker layers also mean that more aggressive scrubbing will be needed. Fortunately, with salt scrubs, it's possible to remove even the most stubborn layers and still have perfectly moisturized skin.

Better Hygiene

Salt scrubs also strip the skin of any excess oils and bacteria by removing the dead layers, effectively unclogging the pores.

Without clean pores, your skin can't breathe, but by using these scrubs, you won't have to worry about any razor bumps or ingrown hairs, which are typically caused by bacteria getting into the open follicles after shaving or waxing. Since foul smells after sweating are caused by microbial activity, reducing the number of bacteria also allows you to keep your skin smelling fresh between cleansings. Keeping your skin clean will also prevent it from becoming irritated and itchy from sweating or any environmental factors.

Anti-Inflammatory Effects

Not only do minerals contained in certain salts reduce the number of bacteria, but they are also able to alleviate the symptoms of certain skin conditions. Magnesium, in particular, is one of the most effective components that soaks the liquid that's building around the inflamed area, reducing the swelling and the painfulness of the skin. The highest amount of magnesium is contained in Epsom salts, alongside sulfates, which help carry away the toxins the bacteria has released with the skin. These toxins are typically responsible for itching as well, which means eliminating them comes with instant relief.

Full Body Invigoration

When you are exfoliating with salt scrubs, you are massaging your skin with an abrasive substance, which significantly increases capillary circulation. The higher the level of friction is between the particles and your body, the more noticeable the results will be. The skin will instantly have a more natural color and will feel and look plump. If applied regularly, these results will last until the next treatment, and you will feel their effect as well in your entire body. As your circulation improves, you will feel more invigorated and full of energy after your relaxing experience.

Enhanced Regeneration

Stripping away layers of dead skin allows your body to soak up every bit of the moisturizer you use - and not only during exfoliation. While it's true that combining salts with oils is the best way to instantly rehydrate your skin, without those dead cells in the way, your skin will be able to do this afterward as well. Keeping new skin cells moisturized is crucial for their growth, as the appropriate lotion supplies them with water and necessary nutrients as well. This accelerates the regeneration process, which can be helpful for many different skin types - from older, discolored skin to a newly scarred one. Faster cell growth means significant improvement for skin tone and texture, which means that exfoliation with salt scrubs is one of the best ways to achieve a much younger appearance.

Salt Body Scrubs

There are many different types of sea salt scrubs recipes that provide several benefits. Here, you will find five simple, organic formulas you can make any time you feel like pampering your skin.

Ginger and Poppy Seed Salt Scrub

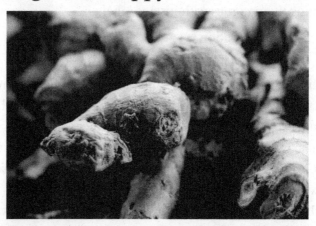

https://unsplash.com/photos/a-close-up-of-a-bunch-of-ginger-roots-Pj8qDxCuMTs

Ginger

The coarse texture of the Himalayan salt is perfect for cleansing your skin and stripping it of all the debris. At the same time, this recipe uses glycerin and Vitamin E – both of which play a huge role in keeping your skin healthy and youthful. And to make the formula even richer, the avocado oil will make sure your skin is plump and nourished. Both poppy seeds and ginger contain powerful antioxidants and can help prevent inflammation and skin irritation.

Ingredients

- Pink Himalayan salt - 1 cup or 280 grams
- Lemon essential oil - 1 tbsp or 15 ml
- Glycerin - 1 tbsp or 15 ml
- Vitamin E - 1 tbsp or 15 ml
- Avocado oil - 2/3 cup or approximately 158 ml
- Poppy seeds - 1 tsp or 9 grams
- Freshly grated ginger - 1 tbsp or 2 grams

Where to Find the Ingredients

Some Ingredients - The pink Himalayan salt, ginger, poppy seeds, and avocado oil - can be found in any supermarket. Lemon essential oil and glycerin are typically sold in beauty supply stores in pharmacies. When it comes to Vitamin E, this recipe works best in topical oil form. However, you may also buy it in an edible tablet form at any supplements store if you find this more convenient.

Directions

1. Place Himalayan Salt in a large bowl and mix it with the freshly grated ginger and the poppy seeds until well combined.

2. Slowly pour in the avocado oil and stir until the oil coats the salt particles evenly.

3. Add in the glycerin and Vitamin E, combining them with salt and oil to reach a spreadable formula.

4. Lastly, when satisfied with the consistency, carefully add the lemon essential oil, and stir the mixture again.

5. You can use this scrub right away or scoop it into a glass container and store it in a cool place for a few weeks.

Rosemary and Lemon Salt Scrub

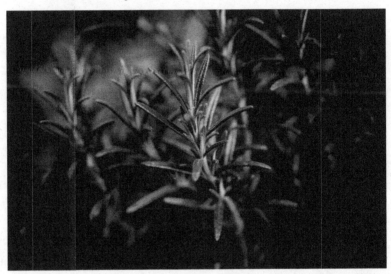

https://unsplash.com/photos/green-plant-in-close-up-photography-Wl-z9lbwkSI

Rosemary

The citric acid in lemon juice is a very powerful natural exfoliant; combined with Epsom salt, it will make sure your skin is appropriately cleansed. Since it also contains a double dose of rosemary, this recipe is ideal for sensitive skin. The soothing properties of this plant perfectly counteract the abrasiveness of the salt, preventing any symptoms of irritation the scrubbing would cause.

Ingredients

- Coconut oil - 2 cups or 473 ml
- Epsom salt - 1 cup or 236 grams

- Rosemary essential oil - 15 drops or 0.75 ml

- Fresh rosemary - 1 tbsp or 2 grams

- Lemon juice - from 1/2 lemon

Where to Find the Ingredients

You will find lemons and rosemary in the fresh produce section of your local supermarket. Make sure they are pesticide-free so that they are safe to apply to your skin. Rosemary essential oil is sold in beauty supply stores or pharmacies, along with Epsom salts.

Directions

1. Finely chop the rosemary just before preparing the scrub, so it would still be fragrant. Soften the coconut oil in the microwave in the meantime.

2. In a large bowl, pour in the Epsom salts and the coconut oil and mix the two until you see that the oil coats the salt evenly.

3. Start adding the rosemary essential oil very slowly, ensuring you don't add too much. It's a very fragrant oil, so the indicated amount is more than enough.

4. Finally, stir in the chopped rosemary and the lemon juice when your mixture is already homogenous and spreadable.

5. Due to the fresh rosemary, it's best to use this scrub right away before this ingredient loses its potency.

Almond Lavender Sea Salt Scrub

If you are looking for a scrub that will help you relax while exfoliating, lavender will accomplish that. It can be very beneficial during dull winter months when you need a gentle antibacterial cleansing and to calm your senses while waiting for spring to come. The sweet almond oil in this recipe acts like a rich, organic moisturizer reducing any damages caused by the sun, natural aging, or inflammatory skin conditions.

Ingredients

- Sea salt - 1/2 cup or 250 grams (for fine grind)
- Sweet almond oil - 1/3 cup or approximately 80 ml
- Dried lavender blossoms - 1 tbsp or 3 grams

Where to Find the Ingredients

All the ingredients of this recipe can be acquired in health food or supplement stores. Sea salt can also be found in any convenience store, and you can decide how coarse you want it to be. However, since it's also combined with herbal exfoliants, you may want to use a finer grit.

Directions

1. First, grind the lavender blossoms until you get a similar texture to salt granules.

2. Mix the sea salt and the ground blossom until well combined, then add in the sweet almond oil.

3. The almond will determine the thickness of the formula, so be careful when adding.

4. When you are satisfied with the consistency of the scrub, it will be ready to use.

5. You can store any leftovers in a cool place for a couple of days.

Grapefruit Salt Scrub

If you need a refreshing formula that, besides exfoliating your skin, also rejuvenates your entire body, a grapefruit salt scrub could just be what you are looking for. The acid in grapefruits effectively strips away all the dead skin cells yet is mild enough to be applied to problematic skin.

The sea salt minerals have anti-inflammatory properties and will help the skin heal. The carrier for this scrub is jojoba oil that soothes irritated skin and reduces any damages caused by environmental factors.

Ingredients

- Sea salt - 1 cup or 220-250 grams depending on the grind

- Jojoba oil -1.5 cup or approximately 350 ml

- Grapefruit zest - from 1 medium grapefruit

Where to Find the Ingredients

The beauty of this recipe is that all of its ingredients can be found in any convenience store. When buying them, make sure they are all organic, paying particular attention to the grapefruit. You will want it to be completely pesticide-free. Whether you use fine or coarse sea salt, it will be up to you - the smaller the grit is, the less abrasive the scrub will be on your skin.

Directions

1. Wash your grapefruit and zest it just before you want to make your scrub. Don't prepare it ahead as it can dry out, losing many of its benefits.

2. In a large mixing bowl, first, combine the sea salt of your choice with the grapefruit zest

3. Start adding jojoba oil in small increments, and continue until you get a paste-like consistency.

4. Use the scrub immediately or within two days. If you have prepared it ahead, keep it refrigerated as it contains fresh fruit.

Clay Sea Salt Body Scrub

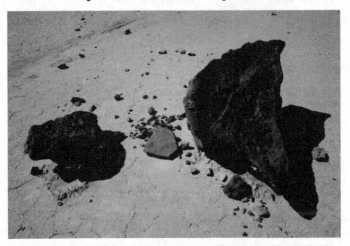

https://unsplash.com/photos/brown-rock-AO3nLHOPf0Q

Sea salt is particularly full of magnesium and calcium - two essential minerals playing significant roles in keeping your skin healthy and polished. Calcium makes sure that the scrub gets into your pores and unclogs them, effectively reducing acne on your body. Magnesium acts as a natural inflammatory agent, which helps keep blemishes at bay. Clay has a very similar effect, and it's also perfect for toning dull, tired, aged-looking skin. The coconut oil nourishes your skin and gives you that healthy, youthful glow.

Ingredients

- Fine sea salt - 5 tbsp or 74 grams
- Coarse sea salt - 5 tbsp or 69 grams
- Bentonite clay - 2 tbsp or approximately 15 grams
- Coconut oil - 2 tbsp or 15 ml
- Lavender essential oil - 20 drops or 1 ml
- Lemon juice - from 1 large lemon

Where to Find the Ingredients

Use extra virgin coconut oil, which you can find in supermarkets or beauty supply stores. Lavender essential oil is typically sold in pharmacies, where you can also ascertain its organic origins. Both coarse and fine salts are available in any well-supplied convenience store - as are organic lemons. Use exclusively food-grade bentonite clay as this is the safest form of organic clay to apply on the skin.

Directions

1. Mix the two types of sea salts in one large bow, then combine them with the clay. Meanwhile, heat up the coconut oil in a microwave for about 45 seconds or until it becomes completely liquid.

2. As soon as the oil is liquified, start pouring it onto the salts and clay mixture while stirring it simultaneously. Make sure the formula looks homogenous before moving on to the next step.

3. Add the lavender oil drops and, finally, when that's also mixed in, squeeze in the lemon juice.

4. Use it right away as a gentle exfoliator, ensuring you don't break the skin in problematic areas because the combination of salts and lemon juice could cause very painful irritation.

5. You can store any leftovers in a glass jar for a couple of weeks.

How to Use Salt Scrubs

Salt body scrubs are the most effective if they are applied to wet, warm skin. For a full spa experience, you may want to take a relaxing bath before exfoliating. Plus, since they are coarser than other abrasives, they need more time to dissolve - but the warmer your skin is, the faster this will happen. Even if you don't have enough time to soak your skin, you should at least take a long shower to open up those pores before applying a salt scrub. Whether you are taking a bath or shower, make sure the doors are closed so the steam can fill the space and remain in the air keeping your skin moist while you apply the scrub.

When applying a salt scrub, always take small dollops and massage them into your skin with your hands or using a mitt. Circular motion works best for reaching all the layers of your skin, especially if you want to exfoliate areas like the elbows and heels, where the skin is naturally thicker. Make sure you scrub one area for around 30 seconds before moving on to the next one. Continue until you have exfoliated all the desired areas of your body, then wash everything off with water. Since wet salt tends to stick to your skin (particularly when combined with a highly moisturizing oil), it's better to wash it away by wiping your body down under lukewarm, running water. When every salt particle is washed off, pat yourself dry with a towel. Don't rub your skin dry, as this may strip away the essential oils that remain from the scrub. Depending on what formula you have used, exfoliating with salt scrubs may require you to use a rich moisturizing lotion afterward. Nonetheless, your skin can only benefit from additional moisture, whether you have used a more aggressive formula or not.

You may use salt body scrubs up to 3 times a week, depending on your skin type and its current conditions. If your skin is on the drier side, it's not a good idea to use it more than once a week, while for people with oily skin, more frequent use is recommended. Regardless of the frequency, if you are using a formula that allows you to prepare it beforehand and store it for longer periods, make sure you mix it again right before you apply it to your skin. After only a couple of hours, the oils and salts in the scrubs tend to separate, and you need them to act together. If you keep your scrubs refrigerated, take them out of the fridge a couple of hours before application because a room temperature scrub is far easier to apply.

Warnings and Disclaimers

While salt scrubs may seem like the perfect natural solution for a home spa night, keep in mind that they can be just as abrasive as some chemical cleaners. Regardless of their grit, salt particles have a particular shape to them, which results in a lot of friction between them and your skin. For this reason, it's never a good idea to use them more than 2-3 times a week, even on oily skin. When used with normal frequency, the minerals in the salt take away just the right amount of excess oil, so your skin will only have a healthy glow but won't appear sweaty. However, applying them too often will strip too much natural oil, which only prompts your glands to produce more sebum. As a result of this, your skin can become very uneven - on some areas painfully dry, while on others terribly oily.

Unless your skin is overly sensitive, applying salt scrubs with rich carrier oils can be beneficial for it - as long as you don't do it too often. Otherwise, your skin will become irritated, cracked, painful, and can even show signs of premature aging. It may take some trial and error to find the best scrub and frequency of application that works for your body. However, you must understand that salts aren't meant to be used as a part of your daily beauty routine, no matter how relaxing or invigorating they may be. The key is to find a balance between what's good for your skin and effective exfoliation.

Don't use salt scrubs on irritated skin, particularly if you have severe, bleeding acne or small wounds from eczema or similar conditions. It's also not recommended to apply it after sunbathing or waxing, as your skin tends to be sensitive after either of those. Apart from causing pain when entering these small cuts, salt can cause further irritation making the tissue swell even more. While some smaller grits may be gentler on the skin, most salt scrubs aren't suitable for facial use either. The skin on your face is the most exposed to all the environmental factors. Therefore, it's usually more sensitive than on the rest of your body. If you also regularly apply heavy makeup, this alone can strip away a lot of moisture from your skin. So, it's best to use an exfoliant that won't dry out your face even more.

Chapter 7: Sugar Body Scrubs

Sugar scrubs are among the most popular natural body exfoliants because sugar is a very gentle yet effective ingredient. As you probably already know, these scrubs are made with sugar granules that can help you mechanically exfoliate your skin and get rid of dead skin and dirt buildup. According to the American Academy of Dermatology, exfoliating with a sugar scrub helps remove the top layer of skin cells, which aids in the removal of excess oils, dirt, and impurities. This leaves the skin glowing and looking smoother. Although they're relatively gentle exfoliants, they shouldn't be used daily. If you're using facial sugar scrubs, it's better to use them a maximum of two to three times a week. If you have sensitive skin, you may want to stick to exfoliating only once per week. If you want to use them for your body, which is the main focus of this chapter, it's recommended that you use them 2 to 3 times per week if you have normal skin. If your skin is oily, you can use sugar scrubs on your body 3 to 4 times a week. If you have sensitive skin, 1 or 2 times per week is enough.

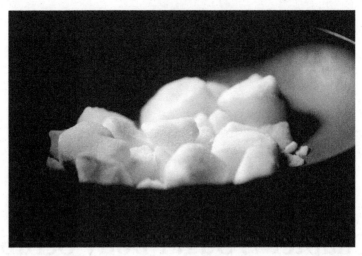

https://unsplash.com/photos/white-sugar-cubes-in-black-bowl-iEqSPa-hNfk

Sugar is generally an excellent skincare ingredient and is used in a wide array of homemade and commercial products. Just about any skincare product that vows to leave your face rejuvenated likely contains a lot of sugar derivatives. Whether it's in its granulated form or an extract, sugar can deliver a wide array of beautifying benefits. For one, it can help lock in moisture as it's a natural humectant. Sugar draws in moisture from the surrounding environment and helps preserve the moisture that the skin absorbs. Products that include sugar and its offshoots substantially refresh the skin's complexion and ensure that the skin remains plump and smooth by locking the moisture into the skin. This can give the illusion of a youthful complexion while fighting against water loss in one's skin. The molecules can aid in soothing and calming the skin. Sugar can unclog the pores and generate a livelier complexion when used in skincare.

Glycolic acid is among the main components of sugar. If you generally read a lot about skincare and are up to date on the latest beauty trends, then you must know how popular it is nowadays. Glycolic acid is an incredible skin brightener and exfoliator. People with uneven skin tones, rough skin texture, acne, hyperpigmentation, and scarring are likely to include this chemical in their routine. Glycolic acid, alternatively known as

AHA or Alpha-Hydroxy Acid, works by penetrating the skin and breaking down the bonds that hold the skin cells together. This phenomenon promotes skin cell turnover, which leaves the skin even-looking and glowing.

In this chapter, we will explore the uses of sugar body scrubs. You will come across various easy homemade scrub recipes that use sugar as a base. There are endless options when it comes to making a sugar body scrub. It can target various skin problems and provide a wide array of benefits, depending on the ingredients you combine sugar with. To ensure that you use these scrubs safely and reap the benefits of all the ingredients, we have included some recommendations regarding usage and after-care precautions in this chapter.

How to Use a Sugar Scrub

Using sugar scrubs is as easy as it sounds. Some people apply their sugar scrub before they hop into the shower, while others do it once they're already inside. It's a matter of preference, though it's best to use it on damp skin. So, if you're toward the end of your shower, use a towel to pat your skin, leaving it a little damp. You need to grab a generous amount of the scrub on your hands and massage it gently into your skin for the best results. You can either use back and forth stroking or circular motions. If some parts of your skin seem rougher than the rest, you should pay extra attention to those areas. These are typically the soles of your feet, elbows, ankles, and knees. These parts of the body tend to harbor dead skin, which makes them in need of a good exfoliation session every now and then. Some people would rather use a hand mitt or a washcloth to apply and massage the sugar scrub onto their skin. It doesn't really matter which method you decide to use as long as you don't press really hard as you exfoliate with the sugar scrub. Sugar particles are already abrasive and rough. If paired with aggressive motion, you can easily damage your skin's protective barrier, promote breakage, and irritate your skin. Be gentle, and the sugar's somewhat harsh nature will do an immaculate job on its own.

You shouldn't wash off the sugar scrub as soon as you apply it; this is a mistake that most people make. Instead, let it sit onto your skin for a while. This allows your skin to benefit from the accompanying ingredients, such as essential oils, which are typically abundant in nutrients and antioxidants and allows the sugar to act as a humectant and entrap the moisture that your skin absorbs. Afterward, you can just rinse the scrub off and enjoy your newly soft and supple skin. You can do this step toward the end of your shower or before you start shaving. Using a sugar scrub to prep your skin before shaving can help unclog pores and get rid of dirt and excess oils, which would help you shave more effectively. This can also help you avoid strawberry legs and ingrown hairs. If you're using a sugar scrub as part of your skincare routine, and not necessarily because you're going to shave, you may want to follow up the process with a good cleanser. If you don't mind the feel of oil on your skin, you can skip this step. It's nice to let the oil sink into your skin throughout the day, providing extra softness and moisture. However, many people dislike the heavy feel of the oil and prefer to wash it off. There is no right or wrong way to do it. It depends on your skin type and what you feel comfortable with. If you like bathing, you can soak in your tub for at least 20 minutes to soften your skin's outer layers. This makes it easier for you to exfoliate and enhances the effects of the scrub.

Besides extending the lifetime of your self-made or natural tan, using sugar scrub a day prior to your spray tan or applying a fake tan at home can help you diminish the risk of having streaks, splotches, and uneven areas or fading.

Types of Sugar You Can Use

There are generally three types of sugar that you can incorporate into your sugar body scrubs. Most people frequently use cane sugar in their recipes and resort to brown sugar as an alternative or whenever they'd like to change things up. However, it's advised that you try all three types of sugar to find out which one(s) work best for your skin.

Brown sugar is the gentlest and least abrasive of all three types, making it ideal for individuals with sensitive skin. They are also the best when it comes to facial scrub recipes. Since it's the least harsh, it may be used up to four times a week, though, as we mentioned, you should still be aware of your skin condition to ensure that you're not going overboard with the exfoliation. Some people may only need to use the scrub once a week, while others can comfortably use it up to four times per week. Pure cane sugar, which is alternatively known as unrefined white sugar, is a great choice for all skin types. It also possesses nutrients that can be quite beneficial for the skin. This type of sugar is more abrasive than brown sugar and should therefore be used not more than two to three times a week. Finally, turbinado sugar or raw sugar is the coarsest and most abrasive of the three types of sugar. This is because it has large granules, making it the ideal choice for body scrubs. It is also the least processed among the three, which is perhaps the reason why it has the highest mineral content. Body scrubs that use this type of sugar as their base should be used up to only two times a week.

Most people stick to olive, coconut, and jojoba oils when it's time to make a homemade scrub. They often forget that nature has countless essential oils to offer – each with its unique properties that can benefit your skin in different ways. You can also use apricot oil, hazelnut oil, avocado oil, hemp seed oil, sesame oil, walnut oil, and sweet almond oil to make your sugar body scrub. Fortunately, since these scrubs are typically free of water content, you don't need to add a preservative to keep them from going bad.

Lavender Sugar Body Scrub

The lavender sugar body scrub will leave your skin looking healthy and vivacious. Aside from its incredible smell, lavender is enriched with anti-inflammatory properties that help nourish and soothe the skin, making it especially helpful for individuals who have dry skin. These antioxidants are also essential because they help protect the skin from damages caused by free radicals. Its anti-inflammatory and antioxidant properties make it perfect for treating sunburns and aiding with psoriasis and eczema. The lavender essential oil also has a calming effect which people who struggle with anxiety may find helpful.

Ingredients

- Your choice of sugar - 2 cups
- Lavender essential oil - 20 to 25 drops
- Coconut oil - 1/2 cup
- Lavender buds - 2 tsp(optional)
- Vitamin E - 1/2 tsp (optional)
- Lavender mica powder - 1/4 tsp (optional)

To make the scrub, choose the type of sugar that's most suitable for your skin type. We recommend adding a carrier oil (fractionated coconut oil) and vitamin E in all your scrubs, along with the initial essential oil. The fractionated carrier oil is lightweight and hydrating. It will leave your skin feeling silky and glow-looking. Vitamin E will help nourish and revitalize your skin. While you don't necessarily need a preservative, vitamin E can keep the carrier oil from oxidizing.

Directions

1. Microwave your coconut oil to ensure correct measurements and ease of use.

2. Combine your sugar and coconut oil, and make sure to mix well.

3. Add your vitamin E and essential oil into the mixing bowl or jar.

4. You can use mica powder to get the lavender color of the scrub. While it's not crucial, your scrub will take after the white color of the coconut oil without the colorant.

5. You can add dried lavender buds for extra exfoliation and a pretty aesthetic if you want.

6. Mix well until all your ingredients combine and hold up like a paste.

Rose Sugar Body Scrub

There is nothing better than exfoliating with an all-rose scrub. This scrub's main ingredient is rose otto, making the skin feel fresh and smooth. Adding crushed rose petals can also make your scrub look more luxurious. Rose essential oil is nourished with antibacterial properties, making it great for anyone who struggles with acne as it helps ward off the bacteria that trigger this skin condition. It also has high antioxidant and anti-inflammatory properties, making it an effective anti-aging ingredient. Like lavender oil, rose essential oil can help diminish symptoms of anxiety and stress and enhance our general well-being. You will undoubtedly feel refreshed after using this scrub.

Ingredients

- Your choice of sugar - 1 cup

- Rose otto essential oil - 20 to 25 drops of rosewater - 2 tbsp

- Coconut oil - 3 tbs

- Pink rose petals - 2 tsp (optional)

- Vitamin E - 1/2 tsp (optional)

- Pink mica powder - 1/4 tsp (optional)

Directions

1. Drop-in, your choice of sugar and dried or fresh rose petals into a food processor.

2. Keep blending until the ingredients are well-combined.

3. The pink rose petals are supposed to give you a pinkish tone, but if you're opting for stronger color, you'll have to add pink mica powder.

4. Use the rose otto essential oil to give the scrub a wonderful scent. Alternatively, you can use 2 tablespoons of rosewater. Since water is an obvious constituent of rosewater, you will have to either use your product quickly or a preservative to ensure it doesn't go rancid. (In this case, you will need vitamin E.)

5. Add Vitamin E.

6. Mix well until your scrub is seamlessly blended.

Lemon Sugar Body Scrub

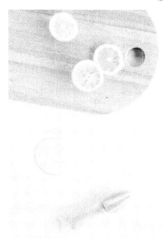

This is the perfect scrub for the summertime. It is quite refreshing and reinvigorating. This zesty scrub can help brighten your skin and leave it feeling silky, supple, and soft. It will give you an incredible glow and is especially suitable for normal to dry skin types. Lemon, when used in a scrub, acts as a great exfoliator. It can also cleanse your skin, nourish it, and rid it of imperfections and problems like excess oil and acne. Lemon, a brightening agent, can help even out and lighten the skin tone. The lemony scent can boost one's energy and improve one's mood.

Ingredients

- Your choice of sugar - 1 cup

- Steam-distilled lemon essential oil/ lemon extract - 20 to 25 drops

- Coconut oil - 1/4 cup

- Vitamin E - 1/2 tsp (optional)

- Lemon zest from one lemon.

Directions

1. To make the scrub, you need to grate an organic lemon to extract the zest and mix it with your desired choice of sugar.

2. Then, combine your ingredients with steam-distilled lemon essential oil/lemon extract, contributing to the wonderful smell.

3. Add your choice of additional essential oil (if desired), your carrier oil, and vitamin E.

4. Mix all your ingredients very well.

Vanilla Sugar Body Scrub

Whether in the form of a cookie, sundae, milkshake, perfume, or body scrub, vanilla is always a lovely treat for the body. The scent of vanilla is warm, welcoming, familiar, and comforting. Combining vanilla seeds with raw cane sugar can make for an amazing and gentle yet effective exfoliant. The added coconut oil creates a soft blend and acts as a conditioning and softening agent for the skin. You'll barely ever come across someone who doesn't favor the scent of vanilla. Aside from the scent, vanilla has antioxidant properties that can help prevent the damage that free radicals can cause. It is also believed to soothe inflammation and can help with anti-aging.

Ingredients

- Raw cane sugar - 3 cups
- Vanilla oleoresin or vanilla extract - 1 tsp
- Coconut oil - 1/2 cup
- Vanilla bean seeds from 1 vanilla bean
- Vitamin E - 1/2 tsp (optional)

Directions

1. Split open the vanilla bean and take out the small black seeds.

2. Mix cane sugar with fresh vanilla bean seeds and add vanilla oleoresin (you can use vanilla extract as an alternative).

3. Add the coconut oil.

4. Mix all your ingredients well.

5. The longer you let the scrub sit, the more prominent its scent.

Mint Sugar Body Scrub

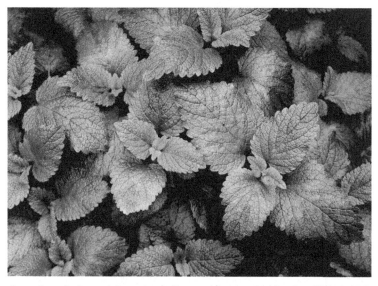

https://unsplash.com/photos/green-leaves-with-water-droplets-boadZKqd1YM

Mint is known for its refreshing properties, and it is also the perfect ingredient for getting rid of dead skin cells. This scrub's texture and the properties of menthol will leave your face refined and plump. Incorporating this scrub into your morning routine will surely help you start your day on an energized note. Mint is known for its unmatchable cool feeling. It is also great at soothing itchy and dry skin. Mint is enriched with antifungal and antimicrobial properties, making it highly suitable for individuals with acne-prone skin. Peppermint essential oil can help unclog pores and regulate excess oils in the skin.

Ingredients

- Your choice of sugar - 1/4 cup
- Coconut oil - 1/2 cup
- fresh/dried mint - 2 tbsp
- Vitamin E - 1/2 tsp (optional)
- Peppermint/spearmint essential oil- 20 to 25 drops
- Green mica powder - 1/4 tsp (optional)

Directions

1. You need to use dried or fresh mint leaves to make the scrub. This will give it its greenish tone and the fresh minty scent.

2. Add the leaves to your carrier oil and vitamin E and mix well.

3. You can typically use peppermint essential oil to give your scrub a minty smell. However, if you have sensitive skin, you may want to use spearmint essential oil instead. You can also use peppermint extract. You need to keep in mind that it won't contain the same beneficial properties as the essential oil.

4. As you know, if you want a more prominent green color, use green mica powder.

Coffee Sugar Body Scrub

If you love coffee, you will certainly love this scrub. Every coffee person knows how stimulating the smell of coffee can be. This revitalizing coffee sugar scrub, enhanced with essential oils, will soften your skin and keep it nourished. The coffee sugar body scrub consists of brown sugar and coffee grounds to make your skin feel soft and silky. The added coconut oil can also help repair your skin's barrier, leaving it feeling supple. Coffee grounds serve as gentle exfoliants. This scrub is rich in nutrients and antioxidants and can therefore balance and regulate the pH levels in the skin. It can also help to diminish the appearance of acne, stretch marks, and cellulite and remove any unwanted tan. Coffee can also boost collagen levels in the skin, which can help diminish the process of premature cell growth. Coffee grounds can also help stimulate blood flow.

Ingredients

- Your choice of sugar - 1/2 cup

- Coconut oil/almond oil - 1/2 cup

- Vitamin E - 1/2 tsp (optional)

- Vanilla essential oil - 20 to 25 drops (optional)

- Ground coffee - 1 cup

Directions

1. If you want, you can use used coffee grounds for the scrub. However, it's better to use freshly ground coffee for the best results.

2. Add the coffee grounds and the sugar to the carrier oil.

3. Mix well.

4. The scent of the coffee scrub is mild. If you want to mix things up, add 20 to 25 drops of vanilla extract or some vanilla oleoresin to make things interesting. You can also add vitamin E for its added value.

5. Stir all the ingredients well to create the final product.

Disclaimers

You should never use sugar body scrubs every day. The recommended number of uses per week can differ greatly from one person to the other. While these numbers are a general rule, you should experiment to find out what feels best for your skin. For instance, one person may feel fine using cane sugar scrubs four times a week, while another person's skin may grow sensitive after just the second use. In this case, they may want to switch to brown sugar or space out the duration between each use and the other. You should never use a scrub on sunburnt or wounded skin. If you know that your skin is incredibly sensitive, avoid using scrubs altogether. You shouldn't use sugar scrubs after getting a chemical peel or cosmetic or medical surgeries. Allow your body to recover from whatever incident or situation it has been exposed to before imposing a harsh scrub on it, as this can hinder the healing process.

When used before shaving, sugar scrubs can also help you prevent the growth of ingrown hairs. Sugar scrubs can aid in the removal of toxins that accumulate as a result of pollution, UV rays, and pesticides. They can remove rough patches on the skin, and if done before tanning (whether it's a real suntan or a fake one), you can make your tan last longer. By exfoliating, you can increase and stimulate blood circulation, reduce feelings of anxiety and stress and tone your skin.

Chapter 8: Body Scrubs with Other Exfoliants

From manicures and make-up to haircuts and facials, Byrdie.com explains that, on average, a woman spends $313 per month or $3756 each year on maintaining and beautifying her appearance. This adds up to $225,360 over a lifetime. Men spend $244 each month on their appearance, adding up to $175,680 each year. Surprisingly, most of that money goes toward facial moisturizing products. They spend the rest of their money on gym memberships, shaving products, supplements, and hand creams. Another study on foxbusiness.com suggests that Americans spend about $15000 on skincare products throughout their lifetimes.

We've heard it all; salicylic acid, niacin amide, AHAs, BHAs, hyaluronic acid, and endless other chemical products. These are all chemicals that undoubtedly do wonders for the skin. Unfortunately, they are often formulated by high-end brands and sold in luxurious packaging. While it's possible, it's not always easy to make homemade salicylic acid and hyaluronic acid serums; you'd have to acquire the chemical powders and turn your kitchen into a mini-lab to get the job done. The consistencies and constituents of chemical formulas are also not to be played with. The tiniest mistakes can result in grave consequences. While leaving the chemical formulas to the experts makes more sense, replacing the empty products on your vanity every other month can break the bank.

Earth is a vast place, offering endless resources that prove beneficial for our health, whether they are to be used topically or consumed orally. We are often fixated on the wide array of essential oils, ranging from jojoba and sweet almond to hibiscus and lavender oils, forgetting that there's more to nature's incredible healing and rejuvenating agents than just these natural products. While essential oils offer indispensable benefits for our skin's health, mindfulness, and peace of mind and play great roles in our daily skincare routines, we should still explore other less common organic skincare alternatives. Homemade scrubs are not limited to popular natural ingredients like oils, coffee, salt, oatmeal, and sugar explored throughout the previous chapters. You may be surprised to learn that almost anything natural and contains beneficial properties of some kind can be used in a body scrub.

Our skin functions better when it's clean. You can't expect to benefit from overly expensive creams, moisturizers, and serums when you have dead skin, product, and dirt buildup. Regular exfoliation is needed to maintain your skin and keep it clean. However, you can't rely solely on abrasive scrubs like those containing sugar, coffee, and salt granules, as they can't be used daily. People with sensitive skin may not be able to use these types of scrubs more than once or twice a week. With that being said, nature offers numerous other ingredients that aren't as abrasive and can be used more frequently.

This chapter will explore other unconventional scrub ingredients that can be used for the skin. Chances are, you will find most of the ingredients lying around your kitchen or hidden deep inside one of your cupboards. You'll find out how you can make beneficial scrubs with easy-to-find ingredients at home.

You'll also understand what each of them is used for and how it can help rejuvenate your skin.

Best Practices

You can help maintain your skin's circulation and general health by using scrubs daily. However, as we mentioned, using scrubs that contain abrasive granules like salt and sugar every day can cause skin breakage and harm you in several ways. If you think about it, your skin serves as a barrier between your body and all the harmful external conditions. It keeps our tissues and organs protected and safe from potential infections and damage. It also helps retain body fluids, prevents water loss, and keeps our body temperature regulated.

Your skin deserves the type of care that it gives the rest of your body. You also need to take care of it to help it carry out its job and ensure that it functions efficiently. The skin is so much more than our general appearance. Impurities and skin conditions often suggest that there may be something wrong with the way your body is functioning. By using scrubs, you encourage your skin to shed dead cells, flush out harmful toxins, and release fluid retention in the body. Besides these general health benefits, each ingredient that you include in your recipe offers a unique advantage. In most cases, or when done right, the scrub will reveal glowing and smooth skin. You can follow the exfoliation process with a wrap, sauna, or steam to rejuvenate and revitalize your skin.

During the scrub, the nutrients and health benefits derived from whichever ingredients you're using can help stimulate your skin's metabolism and promote the oxygenation of cells. As you probably already know, Asia is home to the best natural ingredients you can find, and they have the best skin scrubs and remedies. In India, for instance, they follow up a typical oily Ayurvedic treatment with a cleansing paste made of ground lentils, herbs, and flour, known as *ubtan*, to get rid of the excess oil buildup that results from the treatment. In Indonesia, they've been using a ground pumice stone, coffee beans, honey, clay, and coconut for years to exfoliate the skin. Scrubs consisting of rice, honey, and seeds are widely popular across Thailand. They help moisturize, tone the skin, and promote healthy blood circulation. Flour, groundnuts, and similar ingredients are commonly used in Sri Lanka, while exotic Japanese ingredients, like pearl barley powder, black sugar, adzuki beans, soybean flour, rice bran, buckwheat flour, and a wide range of green leaves, vegetables, and fruits are used to make scrubs in Japan. To them, the process of exfoliating the skin and using a cleansing body scrub is just as important as the bath or shower.

You can purchase a useful scrub tool, such as silk mitts, loofah mitts, cotton or waffle hand towels, and natural wood brushes to help you make the most of your exfoliation process. The most important thing is that you use tools that are made of natural fabrics and unbleached wood. We recommend that you use a dry brush each morning and use it to make strokes across your body toward the direction of your heart. While showering or bathing, use the brush to carry out the same motion under cool to warm water. You should stop when your skin turns somewhat pink. Then, fill up a cloth or muslin bag with any of the exfoliating ingredients we mentioned above, such as adzuki bean powder, rice bran, seaweed, or oats, and continue to scrub it onto your skin, under running water, in tiny circular movements. Start at the bottom, from your feet, and start moving up to your legs, your arms, and the rest of your body. After you wash off the body scrub, you can rub aromatherapy oil on your body in strokes toward the direction of your heart.

Alternatively, you can use one or a collection of the natural scrubs that we will recommend throughout the chapter.

Rice Bran Scrub

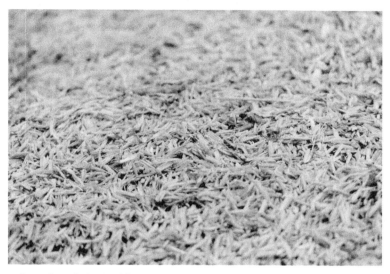

https://unsplash.com/photos/a-close-up-of-a-pile-of-brown-rice-tyVcPQfncrg

Rice bran is a rice grain's outer layer. It is where the grain stores all its vitamins and nutrients. When we eat regular white rice, we don't receive the nutrients held in rice bran, as they're milled and removed. Fortunately, we can purchase rice bran on its own and incorporate it into our baked goods to make them healthier and more enriching. Rice bran is not only known for its nutritional value, however. Japanese women have been using it for centuries to exfoliate and achieve great skin quality. It is a highly esteemed beauty treatment, which is why it is now very popular in different parts of the world and can get quite pricey. Luckily, rice bran scrubs are very easy to make at home.

Ingredients

- Rice bran - 3 tbsp

- Cold milk - 1½ tbsp

- Highly concentrated green tea (many leaves, little water) - 3 tbsp

- /Orange juice - 1½ tsp

- Extra virgin olive oil - 2 tsp

Directions

1. Put all your ingredients in a small bowl.

2. Mix very well until you reach a creamy consistency.

3. To make sure that you can easily spread it on your skin, it shouldn't be too dry or runny.

4. To reach the right consistency, add more rice bran to thicken the paste or add more liquid to water it down.

Make sure that your skin is clean before using this scrub/mask. Apply it onto your body using small, circular motions, and when done, leave it to dry out. This will ensure that your skin has absorbed all the nutrients. Don't walk around with it, as it can crumble and make a mess. Once it dries out, hop into the shower, wet your body (don't wash it off), and rub it in using small circular motions.

Wheat Bran Scrub

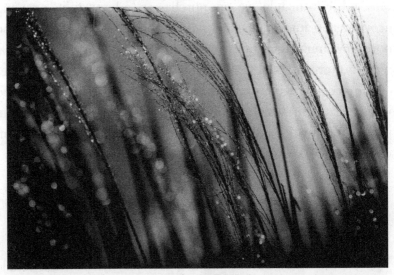

https://unsplash.com/photos/selective-focus-photography-of-brown-grass-at-daytime-uYTKzVp8loQ

Wheat bran can do wonders for the skin. Like rice bran, wheat bran is a wheat grain's outer hard coat. It also stores various beneficial and nourishing agents and properties. For one, wheat bran contains selenium, which serves as an amazing antioxidant, protecting the skin from harmful sunrays and damage. Wheat bran is also enriched with vitamins B and E, which can help rejuvenate the skin. They are gentle cleansers and exfoliators and are quite effective at fighting signs of aging. Wheat bran offers great nourishment and benefits for the skin. The scrub also contains two other prominent ingredients: baking soda and coconut oils. Baking soda is also known as sodium bicarbonate. It is an alkaline chemical formula enriched with antifungal, antibacterial, anti-inflammatory, and antiseptic properties. It's effective at combating pimples and acne, exfoliating the skin, and enhancing your complexion. You are now well-versed in the benefits of coconut oil as an antimicrobial, repairing, moisturizing, and anti-aging agent!

Ingredients

- Wheat bran - 6 tbsp
- Baking soda - 3 tsp
- Coconut oil - 3 tsp
- Water as needed

Directions

1. Put all your ingredients in a clean bowl.

2. Mix everything well.

3. Your consistency needs to be similar to a smooth paste. You can add the necessary amount of water to achieve this texture.

4. Before each use, make sure to add coconut oil to the scrub and mix with water.

5. Some people prefer to use milk instead of coconut oil.

Massage the scrub onto your body for a few minutes. Leave it on for around 5 to 6 minutes for your skin to absorb it. Then, scrub it onto your skin again before finally washing it off. Pat your body dry. This scrub works on moisturizing, exfoliating, polishing, and cleansing the skin effectively. It helps remove dead skin cells and diminish the appearance of tanning.

Walnut Scrub

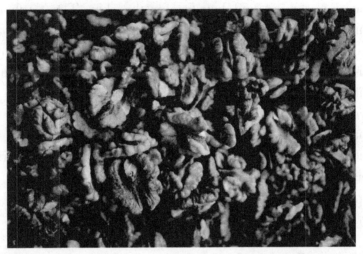

https://unsplash.com/photos/brown-nuts-IbL3Zd62Q7Q

Walnuts are among the best foods for the skin and body. They are enriched with Omega 3 fatty acid, a key component of all our cell walls. Omega 3 is an energy source that ensures your body is functioning as well as it should be. When used in scrubs, Walnuts can help make the skin feel soft and plump. It can also help you get rid of any impurities and toxins. Walnuts are also great humectants. They can aid in retaining moisture in the body so it doesn't become dry. Amla, or Indian gooseberry, can help make your skin softer and firmer. It can promote an increase in vitamin C levels in the skin and boost the production of collagen. Amlas can help in tightening and cleansing your pores, which would make them look smaller. It can generally make your skin look more youthful. Honey is wonderful at lightening scars, fighting off pimples and acne, providing a natural glow, gently exfoliating, cleaning pores, and deep moisturizing.

Ingredients

- Walnut shells - 3 to 4 shells
- Amla - 1 or 2 amlas
- Honey - 1 tbsp

Directions

1. Grind your walnut shells until they're fine, soft particles. Don't aim for a powdery consistency, as you need the granules for the scrub. However, don't leave them large and rough.

2. Mix the honey with the walnut shells to create what looks like a paste.

3. Grind the amlas to make some sort of juice and drop it into the paste.

4. Mix well and pour into a jar. Shelf-life is no longer than a month.

Massage the scrub gently onto your body in circular motions. Scrub your skin for at least 5 minutes, and afterward, leave the scrub on for an additional 2 minutes. This will ensure that your skin absorbs all the benefits of the ingredients. Use lukewarm water to wash the mixture off, and then pat dry. Follow up with a moisturizer to retain moisture.

Buckwheat Honey Scrub

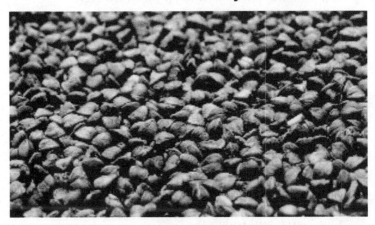

https://pixabay.com/photos/buckwheat-close-up-grains-cereals-3478557/

As we mentioned above, honey has endless benefits to offer. It is classified as a superfood that's enriched with antibacterial, antiviral, and antimicrobial properties. It is also an incredible immunity booster that includes over 200 components, including amino acids, minerals, and enzymes. These are all great benefits for anyone who adds honey to their yogurt, morning oats, and milk. Incorporating buckwheat honey into your beauty and skincare routine can do wonders for the skin. Buckwheat honey typically includes higher amounts of antioxidants, making it an even more helpful component than just purifying and softening the skin.

Ingredients

- Raw buckwheat honey - 6 tbsp
- Fresh lemon juice - 3 tsp
- Brown sugar - 2 tbsp

Directions

1. Put all your ingredients in a bowl.
2. Mix well until your mixture looks like a paste.

Massage the scrub gently onto your skin, allowing it to absorb the moisture. You can leave it on for 5-10 minutes to receive the ultimate benefit of the mixture. Afterward, rinse your skin properly with warm water and moisturize it with your preferred lotion.

Flaxseed Scrub

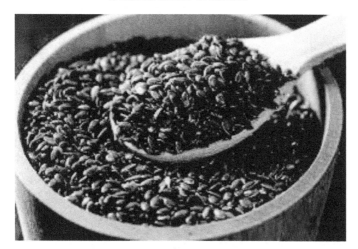

Image by Marco Verch Professional Photographer
https://creativecommons.org/licenses/by/2.0/
https://www.flickr.com/photos/30478819@N08/31558777577

Like walnuts, flaxseeds are quite rich in omega-3 fatty acids. They're also abundant in omega-6 fatty acids. Omega fatty acids can make your skin look younger, revitalized, healthier, and smoother, regardless of its type. They help soften and reinforce the skin's surface and keep the skin hydrated. They can help calm sensitivity, itchiness, and redness and diminish the appearance of dryness and flakiness of the skin. They noticeably protect the skin against signs of external damage and reduce the appearance of fine lines and wrinkles. Flaxseeds also have high antioxidant content and can decrease inflammation. This makes them the perfect natural ingredient for anyone who struggles with psoriasis, acne, rosacea, or dermatitis.

Ingredients

- Flaxseed meal - 4 tbsp

- Raw cane sugar - 8 tsp

- Sweet almond/ coconut/ jojoba/ olive essential oil - 8 tbsp

Directions

1. Drop all your ingredients into a blender and blend well.

2. You can also use your hand. However, a blender can ensure that the flaxseed meal and sugar are seamlessly blended.

Apply the scrub onto your body and scrub lightly in circular motions. Take your time to allow your skin to absorb the oils. Wash off the scrub with lukewarm water. The excess oil can keep your skin hydrated for the rest of the day. However, if you want to get rid of it, use a cleanser to clean it off. Pat your skin dry and follow up with a moisturizer.

Orange Peel Scrub

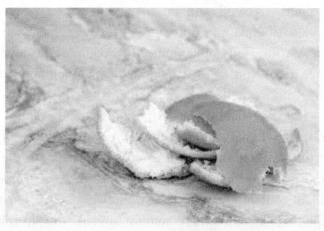

Image by Marco Verch Professional Photographer
https://creativecommons.org/licenses/by/2.0/
https://www.flickr.com/photos/30478819@N08/50635298728

Everyone knows that oranges are fortified with vitamin C. Vitamin C is now among the most popular skincare ingredients. Beauty gurus and aestheticians everywhere are swearing by this incredible agent. Luckily for us, orange peels, which are the main focus of this scrub, are where the most vitamin C can be found. Vitamin C can help boost collagen production in the skin, promoting firmness, hydration, and suppleness. Vitamin C can also aid sunscreen and boost its performance as it can help protect against harmful UV rays. It can also encourage wound healing – beneficial to individuals who struggle with acne. Orange peels also include vitamin A, which encourages skin firmness and softness, helps regulate sebum production, promotes healing, and aids in diminishing the appearance of wrinkles and fine lines. Vitamin B is also a constituent of orange peels. It boosts skin repair and regeneration, promotes skin hydration, promotes a healthy glow, and holds back sebum production. Calcium, which encourages skin hydration and sebum production regulation, can also be found in orange peels. Orange peels also include magnesium which balances hormones that can trigger acne. Finally, it contains copper, which promotes collagen and elastin production, encourages moisture retention, and helps the skin regenerate and fight damage.

Ingredients

- Cane sugar - 1/2 cup
- Dried orange peel - 1 tbsp
- Jojoba essential oil - 2 tbsp
- Sweet orange essential oil - 20 to 25 drops

Directions

1. Put the dried orange peel and the sugar into a bowl.

2. Grab another bowl and combine the jojoba oil with sweet orange essential oil drops.

3. Add the oils into the same bowl as the dried orange peels and the sugar.

4. Stir your mixture well and pour it into a jar to store away.

Take a handful of the scrub and apply it to your skin. Scrub gently in circular motions, and leave the mixture onto your skin for a few minutes. Wash it off and pat your skin dry. Finish off with your preferred moisturizer.

Planet Earth has countless beneficial resources and agents to offer. Organic ingredients can greatly benefit the skin. Instead of spending a fortune on high-end skincare brands, you can use easy-to-find ingredients to make incredible scrubs at home. You always need the right ingredients to create a highly effective body scrub. Many people don't realize that many of these ingredients can be found in most of their pantries or cupboards. This is because as food-grade sources offer nutritional value to our bodies, they are also nutritious for the skin. Organic ingredients are easily absorbed into the skin through its cells. They can help speed up the skin's metabolism, promoting growth and cell turnover and encouraging repair. These scrubs can aid us in detoxifying and cleansing our skin.

Chapter 9: Face Scrubs

Many people underestimate the importance of incorporating exfoliation into their facial skincare routine. If you're on the skin and self-care side of Instagram and TikTok, you must have come across endless posts and videos preaching about the inclusion of toners, ampoules, serums, and peeling solutions in your routine. You are missing out on endless benefits if your facial care regimen lacks frequent exfoliation.

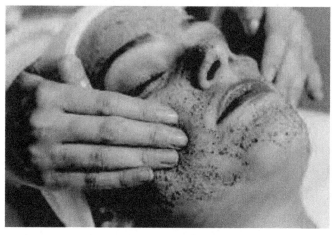

https://pixnio.com/media/pretty-girl-spa-center-massage-face-beautician

Maintaining a healthy skin care routine is not just about following various tiresome steps. You need to ensure that each product you're using has something to offer for your face, targets a certain problem, or maintains a specific condition. Otherwise, the chances are that you'd be bombarding your face with way too many products at once. Not only can this cause irritation and disrupt your skin's protective barrier, but it can also stop your products from working. One product, however, that you surely need in your regimen is a facial scrub. When made using the right ingredients and used correctly, face scrubs can prove to be indispensable. Face scrubs are designed to clean the deep impurities in the skin. They also make your skin glow and brighten up.

Incorrect usage of face scrubs can severely damage the skin and disrupt its outermost protective barrier. Face scrubs are abrasive, which is why harsh usage and excessive pressure can cause breakages and wounds. Before using a face scrub, make sure to wash the skin thoroughly with lukewarm water. For the best results, it's recommended that you use a facial cleanser too. Then, take a nickel-sized amount of your facial scrub and apply it to your wet face. Rub the scrub gently in a circular motion, using your fingers, without applying any pressure. Start at the bottom of your face, going upwards, paying extra to your T-zone area, which includes your forehead, nose, chin, cheeks, and upper lips. Keep massaging your face with the scrub for around 10 to 15 seconds, and then move onto your neck and the exposed area above your chest. Many people neglect these parts when following through with their facial care regimen. Massage this area for 10 seconds and wash your face with cold to lukewarm water after you're done exfoliating. Use a soft towel to pat your face dry and follow up with your favorite moisturizer.

Besides removing dead skin cells and unclogging pores, facial scrubs can help get rid of flakes and lighten acne scars. Exfoliating can also help prevent ingrown hairs, which in turn reduces the development of acne. Facial scrubs can help soften and brighten up the face while improving its texture. Deep cleaning of the face and getting rid of dead skin buildup can allow your skincare products to work better. Impurities can prevent products from being properly absorbed.

In this chapter, you will learn about the difference between facial and body scrubs and why they shouldn't be used interchangeably. You'll also come across facial scrub recipes that target various purposes or issues. Upon reading this chapter, you'll find usage recommendations and after-care precautions.

Body Scrub vs. Face Scrub

When it comes to your face, specializing is key. Many people believe that since facial and body scrubs do the same thing, they can be used interchangeably. They can't possibly be more wrong. Regardless of whether they are intended to be used for the face or the body, Scrubs can help keep the skin clean and radiant. However, we can't use products that can put us at risk of developing rashes, allergies, or breakages, especially in sensitive areas of the body. Our faces are generally very sensitive. Therefore, using body scrubs, typically made of more abrasive and larger particles, can cause great harm. Additionally, body scrubs usually contain perfume, which can be aggressive on the face.

Some ingredients used in body scrubs may not be suitable for certain people. For instance, those with acne-prone skin may be able to use coconut oil-infused body scrubs. However, once used on the face, their skin will break out like never before. The skin on our face is quite different from the skin on our body. While both need to be exfoliated frequently, you will likely never find a product that suits the face and body alike. Body scrubs are generally a lot thicker and have a higher acid concentration than facial scrubs. If you use highly acidic products on your face, you could be putting yourself at risk of acne breakouts and skin irritation.

Acne-Fighting Facial Scrubs

Exfoliation is quite important for acne-prone and oily skin. When you allow dead skin cells to keep hanging around on your face, you're encouraging them to block your pores and make comedones, which are a type of acne blemish often caused by oil and dead skin. Comedones are the starting point or phase of all pimples in the skin. It doesn't matter if you suffer from severe or mild acne. No matter what your skin type is, you can still reap the benefits of facial scrubs. Frequent exfoliation can soften, smoothen, and brighten the skin. The reason why exfoliation is especially beneficial for acne-prone skin is that, as you know, it prevents pus, sebum, and dead skin cells from occupying the pores, clogging them up, and causing breakouts.

Oatmeal Facial Scrub

Oatmeal has endless benefits to offer to the skin. It contains vitamin E, which can promote youthful-looking skin while reducing inflammation. It is also an antioxidant, which can help protect the skin. Oatmeal can also help reduce itching and relieve irritated skin due to its anti-inflammatory properties, making it ideal for acne-prone skin. It's a gentle exfoliator that can help keep the skin safe from harmful UVA rays and other environmental factors. Oatmeal can help improve overall skin complexion, stimulate collagen production in the skin, and absorb excess oil. It is great when it comes to the regulation of sebum production and promoting clearer skin.

Ingredients

- Olive oil - 1 tbsp
- Whole milk - 1 tbsp
- Oatmeal - 2 tbsp
- Rosewater - 6 drops

Directions

1. Mix the olive oil and whole milk in a small bowl.

2. Add the oatmeal to the olive and milk mixture and leave it for a while.

3. After the oatmeal softens in the liquid, add a few drops of rosewater, and stir well.

Gently massage the facial scrub into your skin for 2 to 3 minutes. Rinse with cold to lukewarm water and pat dry.

Honey and Cinnamon Facial Scrub

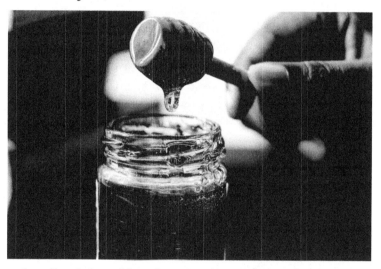

https://unsplash.com/photos/honey-jar-with-honey-comb-yQzrDgU-KAI

Honey and cinnamon are a miracle combination in the skincare world. Not only is it ideal for clearing the pores, but it can also give your skin a glowing appearance. Cinnamon and honey are both fortified with antibacterial properties that can help diminish acne breakouts. They are enriched with anti-inflammatory and antioxidant properties as well, which can help reduce redness, swelling, and itchiness. They can both help protect the skin from harmful environmental conditions and strip the excess oil from the skin. Besides aiding in managing acne breakouts, these ingredients can help diminish black and whiteheads in the skin.

Ingredients

- Raw organic honey - 3 tbsp
- Ground cinnamon powder - 1 tbsp

Directions

1. Mix the honey and cinnamon to create a fine paste.

2. Make sure that the paste is smooth enough so it spreads easily on your skin.

Use a brush to spread the paste evenly onto your skin. Using your fingers, gently rub the scrub in circular movements. Leave the scrub on your skin for around eight minutes to ensure that it absorbs all the benefits that these super ingredients offer. Then, use cold to lukewarm water to wash the scrub off. You can scrub in circular motions once again as you wash the paste off your face. Wash your face using your usual cleanser a few hours later for maximum benefit. To finish off, use a lightweight moisturizer.

Honey, Baking Soda, and Lemon Juice Facial Scrub

Baking soda is a powerful skin exfoliator. It can help eliminate grime, dead skin, dirt, and excess sebum buildups. It deeply cleans skin pores. Lemon juice can decrease sebum production as it serves as a natural antiseptic or astringent.

Ingredients

- Baking soda - 1 tbsp
- Lemon juice - 1 tbsp
- Raw honey - ½ tbsp

Directions

1. Grab a small bowl and add the baking soda and lemon juice.

2. Add the raw honey and mix well to create a paste.

Using the scrub, massage your skin in circular motions for around four minutes. Wash your face with warm water first, and then follow it up with cold water. Use a moisturizer to retain moisture in the skin.

Rice and Honey Scrub

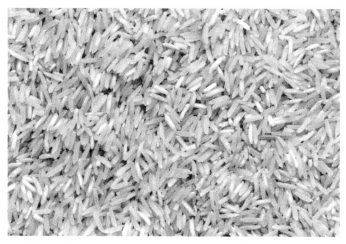

https://unsplash.com/photos/white-rice-grains-on-brown-wooden-table–LdilhDx3sk

Honey can help fade scars, lighten, and brighten the skin, moisturize, heal wounds, and reduce inflammation. Additionally, rice has been a key skincare ingredient in Japan for centuries now. It can help lighten the skin, aid with skin inflammation, reduce blemishes, and promote the production of collagen and elastase. This rejuvenates the skin, makes it appear more youthful and serves as an anti-aging agent. Rice can help promote skin health benefits and eliminate excess oils in the skin.

Ingredients

- Rice- 2 tbsp
- Honey

Directions

1. Grab a small bowl and add the tablespoons of rice.

2. Keep adding honey until you create a thick, smooth paste.

3. The consistency should be even so that the rice particles are still visible and easily felt through the honey.

Cleanse your face with your usual facial cleanser. Leave your skin damp and take some of the scrubs, applying them evenly onto your face. Use your fingers to create light strokes in an upward motion, massaging your face in the process. Leave the scrub on your face for a few minutes before washing it off using lukewarm water. Gently pat your face dry and apply a moisturizer to retain the moisture.

Dry Skin Facial Scrubs

While it may seem counter-intuitive, considering that we explained how exfoliation could strip oils from the skin, you need to use facial scrubs even if you have dry skin. Before you freak out and start visualizing your brittle skin hurting each time you attempt a facial expression or try to form a sentence, remember that there are endless types of facial scrubs and exfoliators – and not all of them cause ill effects. Many people think that exfoliating a dehydrated complexion may result in even more parched skin, resulting in additional irritation. Many people don't know that exfoliation is the key to having moisturized, healthy, plump, and hydrated skin. It's among the few healthy and smart ways to get rid of unappealing flakes on the skin. While there are some ingredients that you should avoid, you shouldn't skip out on the scrubbing and exfoliating process altogether. In all honesty, exfoliating dry skin is not an easy task. One wrong move and your skin can go begging for water! Instead of using mattifying ingredients, seek moisturizing and humidifying agents. Here are some examples of facial scrubs that can aid dry skin.

Green Tea, Sugar, and Honey Facial Scrub

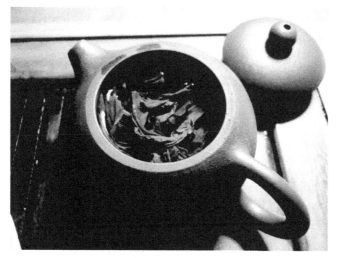

Green tea is an amazing ingredient that's suitable for almost every skin type out there. Unless you're allergic to green tea, it will noticeably improve your skin's complexion. It is among the most popular ingredients in serums, moisturizers, cleansers, spot treatments, and masks. Green tea can help protect the skin against pollution and harmful UV rays. It can also slow down the signs of aging and exhibit soothing effects on the skin. Green tea acts as an active emollient and can help keep the skin hydrated. Sugar is a natural humectant and doesn't draw out moisture from the skin. Honey is also an excellent humectant and retains the moisture in your skin, keeping it supple and smooth.

Ingredients

- Green tea - 7 to 8 bags
- Cane sugar - ½ cup
- Raw honey - 3 tbsp

Directions

1. Cut open your green tea bags and pour the herbs into a small bowl. You can use green tea bags that have already been used as well.

2. Add the sugar into the same bowl, followed by the honey.

3. Mix really well until you are left with a thick paste.

Using your fingers, apply the scrub to your face and rub gently, in circular motions, for around 5 to 6 minutes. While scrubbing, pay extra attention to the dry spots on your face. When done exfoliating, use cold water to wash the scrub off. Pat your skin dry and use a lotion or a serum to moisturize your face.

Honey, Olive Oil, and Brown Sugar Facial Scrub

Olive oil is an incredible natural ingredient for people with dry skin. It is enriched with healthy fats that aid in sealing moisture and protecting the skin. While it aids in moisturizing, it doesn't result in oily skin, as it helps regulate sebum and oil production in the skin. It is also fortified with anti-aging properties and antioxidants. It can maintain the skin's elasticity and firm texture. Olive oil is an exfoliator that removes dead skin cells and promotes glowing skin. Brown sugar is also a natural humectant that helps retain moisture in the skin. The triad could do wonders for dry skin when combined with raw honey.

Ingredients

- Raw honey - 1 tbsp
- Brown sugar - 1 tsp
- Olive oil- 1 tsp

Directions

1. Mix all your ingredients in a small bowl.

2. Stir well until you have a smooth paste.

Use your fingers to scrub the mixture onto your skin. Start from the chin and work your way upward in a circular motion. Keep doing this for around 2 to 3 minutes. When done, use lukewarm water and then follow it up with cold water to close your pores. Gently pat your face dry and apply a moisturizer.

Facial Scrubs for Glowing Skin

Stress and inadequate sleep are recipes for a drab, tired-looking face. Unfortunately, the fast-paced world in which we live today has made it impossible to live without these two factors constantly bugging us out and taking a toll on our appearance. We don't always have the time to wake up extra early to perfect our makeup – and let's be honest, there are days when we wish we could go out without putting on a ton of beautifying products. But when we decide to do so, most of us instantly regret it due to the number of times we hear the words "Are you sick?" Fortunately, there are a ton of natural ingredients that can help bring life back into our faces, rejuvenate our complexion, and achieve a healthy glow. Here are some easy-to-make facial scrubs that can help revive and freshen up our facial skin.

Coffee and Yogurt Facial Scrub

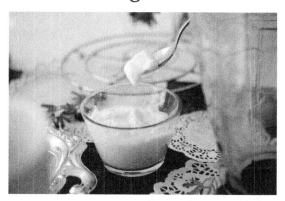

https://unsplash.com/photos/close-up-photo-of-white-cream-in-clear-shot-glass-4calPcmVDII

Caffeine can promote healthy blood circulation and radiant and youthful skin. Coffee is rich in antioxidants, which can help protect us against pollutants, harmful UV rays, and moisture loss. Yogurt is rich in vitamins B2, B5, and B12. It serves as an incredible antioxidant, protecting our skin against free radicals, hydrator, and moisturizers. It is also an anti-inflammatory ingredient. Yogurt is rich in lactic acid, making it an anti-aging agent and an exfoliant that effectively removes dead and dry skin.

Ingredients

- Freshly ground coffee - 3 tsp
- Yogurt/ full-fat milk - ½ cup
- Raw honey - 1 tsp

Directions

1. Mix the freshly ground coffee with the yogurt. If your skin is dry, you may want to replace the yogurt with full-fat milk.

2. Blend your ingredients in a mixer and set aside for a few minutes.

3. Once you can see that your mixture has thickened, add the honey.

4. Mix your ingredients well.

Apply this mixture onto your face and use your fingers to scrub lightly in an upwards circular motion. Do this for 8 to 10 minutes, and then wash it off using cold water.

Coconut Milk and Almond Facial Scrub

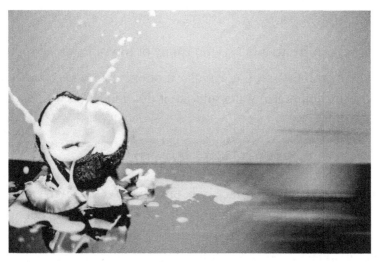

https://unsplash.com/photos/white-and-brown-cake-on-white-ceramic-plate-t_SlQb7j1nE

Coconut milk is a wonderful, gentle exfoliator. It is fortified with high vitamin C content that can maintain the skin's flexibility and elasticity. It can also help prevent wrinkles and fight against skin sagging due to its copper content. Almonds are high in vitamin E, antioxidant, zinc, copper, and Linoleic acid. This makes it an amazing moisturizer, protectant, and promoter of a healthy complexion.

Ingredients

- White clay - 2 cups
- Grounded oats - 1 cup
- Grounded almonds - 4 tbsp
- Finely grounded roses - 2 tbsp
- Coconut milk

Directions

1. Add the white clay, grounded oats, grounded almonds, and finely grounded roses in a bowl.

2. Slowly add coconut milk as you stir your mixture.

3. Add enough coconut milk so it turns into a smooth paste.

4. It shouldn't be too runny or too stiff.

Gently rub the scrub in circular motions onto your skin. Wash it off using lukewarm water and pat it dry. Finish off with a lotion or a serum.

Facial Scrub Best Practices

Start by exfoliating your face only once per week. Then, gradually increase the number of times you use a facial scrub per week until you find the right frequency for your skin type. However, don't exfoliate more than three times a week. If your skin feels irritated, this is a sign that you should decrease the number of times you use a facial scrub or try out different ingredients. Make sure that the ingredients go well with your current skincare regimen. Some chemicals, like retinol, can make your skin very sensitive. This is why you need to make sure that you're using very gentle and moisturizing natural ingredients. You need to choose the right combination of ingredients for your skin type, as well as applying and using the scrub very gently. You don't want to hurt yourself with abrasive particles. Always pat dry your face gently and follow up the process with a lightweight moisturizer that suits your skin type. When applying the moisturizer, you need to make sure that your skin is damp and not completely dry.

Like body scrubs, face scrubs are made to get rid of dead skin cells that accumulate on the surface of the skin. This helps reduce the chances of having your pores clogged and experiencing acne breakouts. Using an exfoliator each week can be your gateway to rejuvenated, healthy, and youthful skin.

Chapter 10: Gifting and Labeling Your Scrubs

Now that you have learned everything that you need to know about homemade body scrubs, their main ingredients, and how to make them, we are going to explain more about storing, packaging, and labeling your new produce.

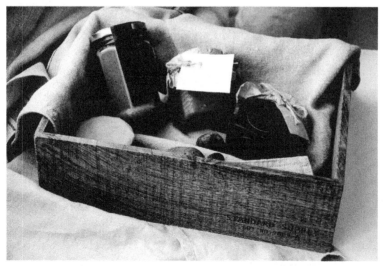

https://unsplash.com/photos/brown-wooden-box-N5fp98wt6h8

How to Store Homemade Body Scrubs

We can't stress enough the importance of properly storing your homemade body scrubs. If you don't, they will go off, and all of your effort and time will be in vain. Usually, homemade body scrubs don't last longer than six months. However, the shelf life may vary depending on the exfoliate you used. For instance, sugar and salt scrubs can last longer, which is why they make great gifts. That being said, make sure you use the body scrub within six months of its manufacture date.

In order to ensure the scrub remains fresh and doesn't go stale, you should store it in a container or jar and make sure that the lid is closed tightly to prevent the carrier oils from going off. However, if the oil goes off, you will be able to tell because you will notice a change in the scrub's smell.

Additionally, the weather that you live in can also contribute to your body scrubs' shelf life. If you live in humid or warm weather, then you should store your homemade body scrub in the fridge. There are some people who recommend that you make the body scrubs into small cubes, put them in an air-tight container, and store them in the fridge so that you can use each one at a time instead of taking the whole container in the bathroom and risk it getting wet or moist. This can make the body scrub last longer.

You are probably wondering why store products last longer than homemade ones? This is because brand products contain chemicals that help extend their expiration date for months or years. Although these chemicals can be safe for use, they can still cause skin irritation, dryness, and allergies for some people. Naturally, you don't want to add any of these chemicals to your natural body scrubs, which is probably why you opted for organic homemade products in the first place. However, there are natural antioxidants that you can add that will help extend the scrub's shelf life, but we will explain them in detail later on.

Now that you have a general idea of how to store your new homemade body scrubs and why it is important to store them properly, let's take a look at a step-by-step storage guide so you can guarantee that your products will last as long as possible.

Use Clean Containers

Making any homemade product takes time, money, and effort, which is why you want to guarantee that it won't go bad in a month or two. In order for your product to have a proper shelf life, you will need to make sure that the tools you use are clean. The containers where you will store the scrub must be clean and sterilized. You should wash them thoroughly using hot water and soap, or just put them in a dishwasher. Even if the containers are brand new, they should still be sterilized. In order to ensure the container is completely disinfected, you should add a little white vinegar during the sterilization process. Unclean jars contain bacteria that can make the oils go bad before their time. Remember to wait until the jars or containers are totally dry before using them. Additionally, make sure that your hands are clean before using the body scrub so that you won't transfer any bacteria to it.

Be Careful with Water

If you are going to use water as an ingredient, then you need to make sure that you only use boiled or distilled water. However, you should wait until it cools down before using it. This will help get rid of any impurities in the water. That being said, using oils instead of water can ensure your product will have a longer shelf life.

Add Antioxidants

If you want your product to have a longer shelf life without using any chemicals or unhealthy ingredients, then you should add natural antioxidants. It is true that antioxidants aren't commonly used to preserve natural products, but they can still give it longer shelf life. This is because they can help by slowing down the oxidation process. Naturally, you will have to open your container every time you use the body scrub, which will expose it and its ingredients to air, which can result in oxidation. There are different types of natural antioxidants that you can use, like rosemary oil or vitamin E oil. These natural oxidants can slow down the oxidation process since they work as natural stabilizers, which will give your product longer shelf life. It is important to note that you shouldn't heat these oils directly.

Storage

Properly storing your homemade body scrub is an essential step to guarantee that it will have a long shelf life. Make sure that the container or jar you use is dark and not clear to protect it from light that can spoil it. Whether you are going to store your body scrub in a clear or dark container, it is essential that you keep the container somewhere dark with a stable temperature. There are ingredients like coconut that can melt, especially during the summer, so it is best to store them in a fridge to guarantee that it lasts for a longer time. Last but not least, make sure that the jar is always covered with a lid and that it is closed tightly to prevent air from getting in.

Remember that every product is different because each has its own ingredients. For this reason, you need to research all of the ingredients that you are going to use and learn about their shelf life and how they will react when mixed. This will help you a lot during the preparation process. You should also know that popper storage and adding certain preservatives can give the product longer shelf life, but it still won't be as long as brand products. However, homemade products are a lot cheaper and healthier, so don't let a short shelf life discourage you. This is why you should only make small amounts to guarantee that they won't go off. If you happen to make more than you need, they can actually make nice and thoughtful gifts to friends and family.

It is recommended that you use the body scrub while it is still fresh because storing organic materials for a long time may make it less effective and lose its texture. This is because some ingredients react badly after being stored for a long time. For example, honey can crystallize. It is better to be safe rather than sorry, so use your homemade body scrub right away while it is still fresh.

Packaging and Gifting

After learning how to make homemade body scrubs, and the correct way to store them so they can have an acceptable shelf life, we will now talk about the packaging. Packaging is a very important step if you are going to gift your product or sell it. As we have mentioned, it isn't recommended to store any organic product for long periods of time because it is better to use it fresh. Therefore, if you are going to make a huge quantity, instead of keeping them until they are no longer useful, you can give them as gifts to your loved ones. Many women, and some men, enjoy using body scrubs, so your loved ones will definitely appreciate the gesture. You can make many and send them as gifts on special occasions like Christmas or birthdays.

Additionally, if you want to make money from your newfound hobby, you can make it a business and sell them online. Online shopping has become so popular, and many people now prefer to use organic products, so you won't struggle to find customers. Additionally, when you give your product to people you know, they can tell their friends about it, and you can start selling it to more people in your circle before expanding. Whether you gift your product or sell it, you will need to package it the right way to create a strong first impression.

How to Package Your Product

When it comes to packaging, it isn't recommended to just pick something fast from the internet. You need to take your time to choose the right packaging for your product. Whether you sell it or gift it, people need to feel that you put a lot of thought into your packaging. Additionally, nice packaging will make people think that the product inside is worth it and is high-quality. They will also be inclined to show it off and display it on social media, which can be a good and free advertisement for your body scrub. Imagine how you feel when you see a product in cheap packaging, you will probably judge it instantly and will feel that it isn't worth your time or money. This is why when choosing a packaging, you should think like the recipient, not the giver. Packaging comes in a wide price range, so whether you have a tight budget or you can splurge, you will be able to find the right packaging for your product.

The first step in choosing a packaging is to pick a theme. Although some businesses seek the help of a graphic designer for this step, you don't need to spend money on outside help as you can do this yourself. Take your time and choose the materials that best showcase your style, personality, and product. However, one thing to keep in mind is to keep it simple. No one wants a package that is too complicated to open or one that has too many colors that can distract from the product.

When choosing a theme for your packaging, there are a few things that you will need to consider first. You need to determine if your packaging should reflect your ethics and values. Like if your product is cruelty-free or eco-friendly, do you want your packaging to reflect that? Or, if you want to show that you care about the environment, in this case, you will have to opt for simple materials and neutral colors. Remember, if you are going to be eco-friendly, then you can't use plastic as it isn't good for the environment.

Additionally, you should ask yourself if you want something extravagant and expensive or if you will opt for something minimalist and more budget-friendly. You should also consider if you are going with something modern or if you feel nostalgic and want to go for something classic. If you want something simple and minimalist, then don't go over the top. Go for something conventional like a simple glass container or jar with a nice drawing or writing on it. Make sure that there is nothing offensive drawn or written on the containers which could be misunderstood so as not to offend people and give the wrong impression. If you are going to sell your product, then ensure your packaging shows professionalism.

If you find it hard to find a theme or feel that you don't know how to create the right packaging for your product, then you can look for inspiration. Go online and research your favorite brands and take a look at their packaging; this can give you an idea of what you want or even what you don't want. Remember not to copy any other brands' packaging, or you will find yourself in legal trouble.

When it comes to containers, yes, aesthetics are important, but so is the product's shelf life. So, as we mentioned earlier, your container must be air-tight so as to not let anything in. Jars and containers come in different shapes and sizes, so pick the ones that best reflect your personal style. You should also pay attention to the lids that you choose. Lids come in various colors and patterns, so choose beautiful and bright colors. There are also lids that have seasonal drawings and patterns on them. For instance, for Christmas, you can opt for lids that have drawings of Santa and snow on them. If you don't want to spend money on glass containers and want a cheaper option, you can use zipper bags.

If you are going to give the body scrub, then consider making the container and packaging customized to the recipients' interests or personalities. This will show them that you care and have put extra thought into their gift.

Labeling

Now that you have chosen a packaging for your homemade body scrub, you will have to label it. As a matter of fact, labeling your finished product is a very important step. If you plan to sell your products, labeling will make it easy for people to recognize it when they see it in a store, and it will make you seem more trustworthy. Additionally, whether the body scrub is a gift or you are selling it, you should include important information about it on the label. Imagine finding a product in a store or being gifted one with no information about the ingredients. Would you still use it? Of course not, because no one will use an unknown product that they know nothing about. This is why you should include all of the ingredients that you used on the label, so people know what they are using. Additionally, labeling can also protect them in case there is an ingredient that they are allergic to, so it could save their lives. Besides ingredients, you should also include the manufacturing date and an estimated shelf life because people would like to know when the product was made and when it will expire. The information that you provide must all be accurate to avoid any awkward situations, or worse, risking someone's life. It is also recommended to include how the product is used. Don't assume that everyone knows how to use body scrubs as maybe they do, maybe they don't, but explaining how it is used can be very helpful, nonetheless.

Gifting

Homemade body scrubs can make for great gifts. Many people are choosing healthier options now, which is why they prefer to use organic products. Gifting your loved ones homemade body scrubs that you made yourself will show them that you care about them and about their health. However, if you are giving a gift, you can't just hand them the container, and you need to put extra thought into it. You should put the body scrub in a gift box, decorate the box from the inside using glitter and small pieces of paper, and on the outside, you can opt for a small ribbon as a decoration. Gift boxes come in different shapes, sizes, and styles, so choose one that will appeal to the recipients. Additionally, if the gift is for an occasion like a birthday or Christmas, then you can choose a box with the appropriate decoration. If you want to make your gift more personal, you can add a personalized note as well. You should also explain to the recipient that homemade body scrubs have short shelf lives and that they should be used right away or ingredients like oils and honey will deteriorate. If you want to give your gift a longer shelf life, then you should opt for exfoliants like sugar or salt, as they can last longer than other ingredients.

Cosmetics Laws and Regulations

Whether you plan to sell or gift your homemade body scrub, there are certain international laws and regulations that you must follow to avoid legal problems. Your ingredients, packaging, and labeling must all follow FDA regulations. For instance, you can't simply put a label on your product that says organic when only one or two of your ingredients are organic. As a matter of fact, a certain percentage of your ingredients need to be organic along with the labeling and handling so your product can qualify for this label. The FDA website will explain the required percentages for organic materials. In addition to that, if you are going to sell your product, then you should make sure to include your business's name and address. The FDA takes labeling regulations very seriously, and this is why you need to be clear on your product's definition. You should also be straightforward and provide accurate information. For instance, you can't claim that your body scrub isn't tested on animals to appeal to people who only use cruelty-free products when your ingredients or the product itself was tested on animals. Additionally, all of the ingredients that you use in your products must be safe and approved by the FDA. You should also provide an expiration date or an estimated product shelf life. However, this information must be accurate and tested to guarantee the safety of those who use it.

Following the FDA cosmetics laws and regulations doesn't only guarantee that the people using your body scrub are safe, but it will also guarantee that you don't get in legal trouble or get sued by a user. For instance, if you use walnut oil and you don't include it in the list of ingredients, and someone with a nut allergy uses your scrub, they may have a severe allergic reaction and sue you and ruin your reputation. To protect yourself and others, before selling or gifting your product, you must do thorough research to have a full understanding of the laws and regulations of the FDA.

Conclusion

From simply keeping your skin healthy and intact to envy-inducing skin rejuvenation, exfoliation can provide you with a large number of benefits. Each one of those could be reason enough to make body scrubbing part of your self-care regime, but boosting your confidence is definitely the best reason to do so. And what better way to become confident about skincare than learning how to make organic exfoliating products you can tailor to the needs of your skin? Yes, there are many commercial products that promise to scrub your skin, unclog your pores, and moisturize your skin to the desired levels. But what if you have all that, without all those other ingredients that store-bought body scrubs contain. Preservatives, emulators, artificial colors, and fragrances have nothing to do with polishing your skin and providing you with a healthy glow.

Fortunately, there is a way to avoid getting all those onto your skin and into your body – exfoliation. Remember, body scrubs remove dead skin cells and unclog your pores, which means that now every substance you come in contact with can enter your skin much more easily. This is one of the main reasons why making and applying only natural body scrubs is so important. There is also the fact that DIY body scrubs can provide you with a relaxing spa-like experience anytime you want it – and for a fraction of the price!

Whether you have used body scrubs before or not, making them will be a whole new, exciting experience. You will dive into the world of textures and fragrances you can safely try on your skin to see their possible effects. This will allow you to determine whether they will make it into your regular skincare routine. Learning how to make your own body scrubs also gives you an opportunity to discover more about your skin. Experimenting with body scrubs means regularly inspecting your skin for any reaction - good or bad. You will be able to notice the subtle changes, which will allow you to adjust the formula until it suits your needs perfectly. And, in case your skin changes again due to environmental factors, you can always make a different natural formula to pamper your skin. This is particularly important for taking care of the skin on your face, which is much more susceptible to irritations and outside factors.

One of the biggest perks of homemade body scrubs is that they are made of everyday ingredients: sugar, salt, coffee, oats, and essential oils – all of which you probably have in your home, whether in the bathroom cabinet or in the pantry. In this book, you were able to find easy-to-follow recipes using these and similar natural types of exfoliants and moisturizers, along with their benefits. Whether you have dry, very dry, sensitive, oily, or combination skin, you will discover a formula that your skin will love. Once you do, the journey towards getting beautiful skin will be much easier. Don't forget to pay attention to the proper application process, and take the necessary precautions afterward, which are equally as important as preparing the perfect batch of body scrub.

Part 2: Body Butters

The Ultimate DIY Guide on How to Make Your Own Natural and Homemade Body Butter, Including Simple and Organic Recipes

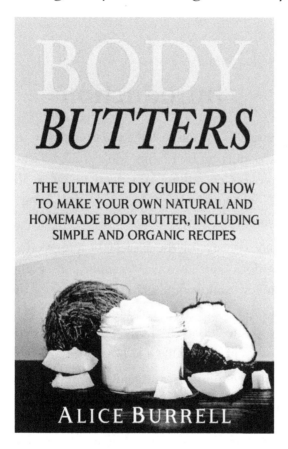

Introduction

Have you always been interested in learning how to make your own beauty products at home but don't know how to get started? This book covers everything you need to know about making natural and homemade body butter by following step-by-step procedures and using simple recipes.

Body butter is one of the easiest beauty products to make because it does not involve complicated equipment and comprises a few simple and natural ingredients. You can get started right away by keeping this book with you as a guide. We will teach you the basics of body butter and mention all the reasons you should be making it at home.

People are becoming increasingly interested in creating their products at home, and it is partly attributed to wanting to use sustainable products with minimum chemicals. While most beauty products are marketed as all-natural and organic, they still contain a few chemicals to help maintain their shelf-life and retain their texture. Once you find out how to create your own body butter, you will realize how easy it is, and you can make a batch that lasts a few months.

Making your own body butter is not only healthier but is also very cost-effective. It is best to buy the main ingredients in bulk so you can make an abundant supply of body butter instead of buying them from the local store. You will soon realize that it costs you a fraction of the price in the long run.

We will discuss the main ingredients for the base of your body butter and what additives to use in your recipes. The book informs you of the various techniques used to combine the different ingredients, and the tools required throughout the process are also mentioned. We will show you how to use essential oils in your body butter, depending on the desired effects of the end product.

In this book, you will learn how to store your products and label them. We will also provide you with step-by-step instructions to use body butter safely, depending on your skin type and needs. Since your product is organic, it needs to be stored and handled in a specific way to make it last longer.

This book also includes a few standard recipes that you can tweak to your liking once you get the hang of the process. You will also find body butter recipes for face masks or moisturizers. Additionally, a few advanced recipes are included for when the basic recipes become too easy for you! This book will become your next best friend as it guides you through experimenting with different body butter recipes, so we encourage you to keep a copy with you and refer to the steps whenever needed. Let's dive deep into the world of body butter and explain how to make them at home.

Chapter 1: Body Butter Basics

You may have come across body butter in the beauty aisle of your local supermarket the last time you went shopping. Are you wondering what this product is? You're in the right place to learn.

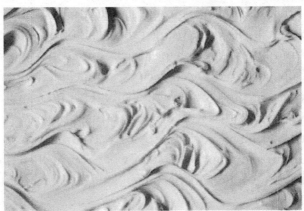

Body butter is essentially a richer alternative to conventional moisturizers and lotions. They are known as "butter" for two reasons:

- They are available in a thick, creamy formulation – reminiscent of the butter you eat.
- Traditionally, they include a "butter" ingredient, namely cocoa butter or shea butter (however, some

modern body butters use coconut oil or vegetable oil and forgo the "butter" ingredient).

Body butter has a long history as a beauty care product.

The History of Shea Butter

Of the most common ingredients used in body butter, shea butter, undoubtedly, has the longest history. This ingredient is derived from the shea tree, which grows in 21 countries across West Africa.

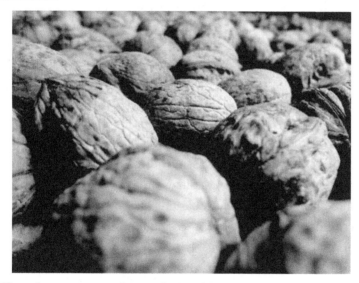

The shea tree produces fruit with a nut inside. The nut is boiled in water, allowing the "butter" to float to the surface. Today, this butter is filtered and processed. However, this butter has been used for much longer than modern production methods.

Anthropological discoveries show that shea butter has been used as a cosmetic ingredient since at least 100 AD. However, there is anecdotal evidence of use that dates even further back. It is said that Cleopatra used so much shea butter as part of her beauty regimen that it was carried to her in large clay pots. Other sources claim that this ingredient was also a staple in the Queen of Sheba's beauty routine.

Research indicates that trade in shea butter dates back at least 4300 years when it was traded in Egypt under King Merenre's rule. Merenre died in 2273 BC, which shows that the use of this beauty ingredient is significantly older than archeological evidence.

The other significant ingredient in body butter, cocoa butter, also has a similarly long history. Cacao beans have been harvested for centuries in West Africa for various reasons, including being the means to create cocoa butter. In this part of the world, cocoa butter was prized for its beauty benefits and also for its culinary uses (it is a significant component of all types of chocolate, including dark chocolate).

In South America, cacao beans were also used for medicinal purposes, including treating uncomfortable skin conditions, burns, and split lips, similar to how it is used today.

The commercial discovery of cocoa butter as we know it today came after the cacao tree was introduced to Europe. Following the growth of interest in chocolate, the cocoa press was invented to make chocolate extraction easier. This process also resulted in the commercial discovery of cocoa butter, leading to further exploration of its benefits by scientists and, ultimately, its widespread use in personal care products today.

Making Your Own Body Butters

The rich history of body butter means there are many recipes available explaining how you can make your homemade and organic body butter.

You may find yourself asking – why? After all, it is relatively easy to pop over to the closest supermarket and pick up a large container of body butter. Additionally, it is unlikely to be overly expensive, depending on the brand.

So, you may wonder why you'd want to go to the trouble of making it yourself.

The answer is relatively simple – chemicals.

Since commercial production is a wide-scale process, companies need to use methods to make their products appealing and have a long shelf life. It means creating body butter that lasts as long as possible and smells better than anything you've smelt before.

This, in turn, means filling their products with numerous synthetic chemicals, including preservatives and parabens, fragrances, and microbeads to add an exfoliating element and more.

Chemicals, in general, are not a bad thing. Everything around you is a chemical. Even the water you drink is a chemical compound of two hydrogen atoms and one oxygen atom. However, the chemicals added to personal care products like body butter during large-scale production aren't as harmless as water.

Many of these chemicals can damage the environment and are directly harmful to you. For example, parabens are thought to disrupt the body's natural hormone function. Though they're "officially" considered safe to use based on EU and FDA regulations, more and more people realize that avoiding these chemicals whenever possible is for the best.

You know precisely what's going into your recipe and on your skin with homemade, organic body butter. You can ensure that you're using only the highest quality ingredients and tailor your recipe to suit your skin type and unique needs.

This last fact is one of the major plus points to making body butter yourself. Suppose you have sensitive skin or are allergic to any ingredients relatively common in popular skincare products. In that case, you know that shopping for commercial products can be a challenging ordeal. It is difficult to find something that meets your needs and, when you do, those products are often prohibitively expensive. Additionally, you're always living in fear that your skin may unexpectedly react to a new ingredient you've never used before or that a trusted brand may have changed its body butter formulation without warning.

Making organic body butter at home ensures you don't have to deal with these concerns. Choosing organic ingredients means that your skin will not react to any traces of herbicides and pesticides which may otherwise be present in the product. Additionally, you can swatch test each ingredient you add to your product, and you will always have control over the formula, meaning you'll never have to deal with the unpleasant surprise of an altered recipe.

Even more promising is that homemade products usually smell much better.

Have you ever wondered why commercial products smell so overwhelming? It is because they need to compete with all the other products on the beauty aisle for your nose's attention. Inevitably, if you have two relatively identical products, you're more likely to go with the one that smells better. It is essential for the manufacturer to produce a body butter scent to entice you to stop in the middle of shopping to try it out.

However, these scents can be much too overwhelming close-up. Remember, your body butter is meant to be a moisturizer. You're also likely wearing a perfume as part of your personal care routine, and you don't want the scent of your body butter to clash with your perfume's fragrance.

By making your own body butter, you can create products that smell fabulous without assaulting all your senses. You can choose a scent that you like and respond to while also opting for one that's subtle enough so that it will not overpower the perfume you choose to wear.

Moreover, with homemade, organic body butter, you can be confident that there are no added synthetic ingredients in the formulation. We already covered parabens and microbeads above, but most personal care products contain various synthetic ingredients that claim to be beneficial for the skin.

However, ample scientific evidence shows that you can receive the same benefits using natural ingredients. Additionally, you may have different opinions about what you apply to your skin. Merely because something's certified as safe doesn't mean everyone will be willing to use it, especially if it is an ingredient harmful to the environment.

By making your own body butter, you have complete control over what is applied to your body. What other people say, or think, is irrelevant. You're free to tailor your recipe to meet your needs and preferences.

Additionally, one of the biggest benefits of producing your products is quality. Even if you're someone who enjoys certain big-name brands and recipes, there's one thing you can't deny, and that is that many of these businesses use minimal quantities of beneficial ingredients like green tea extract and argan oil.

When they use these ingredients in sufficient quantities, there's always a risk they're using low-quality options instead of the best versions possible. The reason is simple – the cost. Businesses can significantly reduce manufacturing costs by skimping on quantity or quality (or both), which has a two-fold benefit. They can sell it to you cheaper, which usually results in higher sales numbers, and they can make more profit on each item sold.

By making your organic body butter, you will always have the confidence of knowing that there's enough of each beneficial ingredient to genuinely help your skin. Additionally, by choosing organic, you know you're only using high-quality ingredients that aren't grown using synthetic hormones and pesticides, meaning that your final product will be of higher quality.

Using **DIY** organic body butter, no matter how you slice it, the benefits are clear. They allow you to have complete control over what you're using on your skin. Remember, your skin is your body's largest organ and will absorb everything you put on it. So, choosing the best ensures that your body is nourished with the proper and healthiest ingredients.

The Benefits of Body Butters

We've discussed body butter and why you should make it yourself using only organic ingredients.

However, you may find yourself asking an even more basic question – why use body butter in the first place? After all, as mentioned above, they're essentially a creamier version of body lotions. So, why not use lotions as you always have? Body butter may indeed be more moisturizing, but can you get the same results by using more lotion?

Not exactly.

Here's the thing about body lotions. Yes, you can increase how much body lotion you use, but you'll need to wait until your skin's absorbed the first application. There's a good chance you'll forget to apply more once the first round dries, which negates the advantage of putting on more lotion.

Additionally, even if you do use more lotion religiously, body butter is simply better at nourishing and hydrating your skin. Body butter generally has richer ingredients than lotions, which is why the difference. So, while you may put on a touch of lotion when you're leaving home or to prep your skin for makeup, body butter plays an entirely different role in your beauty regimen.

The thick creaminess of a body butter clogs your pores, creating a protective barrier over your skin. This barrier reduces the likelihood of atmospheric pollutants like dirt and dust entering your pores and harming your skin.

Some other common benefits of body butter include:

- Smoothens your skin

- Soothes skin conditions like sunburn, rashes, and eczema

- Reduces wrinkles

- Prevents stretch marks and reduces the appearance of existing marks

- Provides your skin with tons of vitamins and antioxidants

- Moisturizes dry, chapped skin and leaves you feeling renewed

But why does body butter offer these benefits?

The science comes down to a single reason – the ingredients.

One thing to keep in mind is that most body butter formulas contain certain fatty acids. Fatty acids like linoleic and oleic acid help hydrate and smooth your skin, and are highly absorbent, so your skin sucks them in quickly. Once inside, they form a protective layer over your skin, which helps keep the moisture inside and provides you with even more hydration. Depending on your formula, this layer can last up to 3 days, providing you with maximum benefits.

These benefits are without even talking about the primary ingredient in most body butter – shea butter.

Shea butter's continued popularity is due to vast skincare benefits. These include:

- High in vitamins A, C, and E

- High in antioxidants that fight off free radical damage and protect your skin from the harmful effects of the sun

- Vitamin A soothes eczema and dermatitis (it is always essential to speak to your dermatologist before starting a new treatment for your skin conditions or discontinuing your existing treatment). Other conditions shea butter can treat include psoriasis, hives, and acne

- Full of healthy fats like omega 3s, which help soothe skin damage, burns, rashes, and more

- Has anti-inflammatory agents that reduce swelling and redness

- Vitamin A also helps with collagen production and rejuvenates your body by prompting your body to replace dead skin cells with new, younger cells.

- Helps soothe itching, which is wonderful for stretching skin. However, it is essential to keep in mind that shea butter will help treat and reduce stretch marks rather than remove them altogether. Depending on the severity of your marks, you may need to speak to a dermatologist for specialist help. In the most severe cases, it is impossible to remove all signs of stretch marks, although Shea butter will help reduce their appearance.

Shea butter, explicitly, and body butter in general, is highly effective on rough skin and when you're looking for a moisturizer for your whole body and not only just your skin. One way to boost the effectiveness of your body butter is to apply it at night before going to bed. While you sleep, your skin is in the repair stage and is, as the name suggests, repairing itself. It is the perfect opportunity for your body butter to work its wonders.

Furthermore, body butter is an excellent option during winter and for people living in dry climates. Your skin dries out due to the climate and can lose essential moisture in these situations. The strong moisturizing properties that body butter offers mean you don't need to deal with the negative repercussions of climatic conditions.

Body Butter in Hair Care

However, these are not the only benefits of good body butter. Many people don't realize that body butter is often a misleading name. While it can be applied to your body, it also has excellent benefits for your hair.

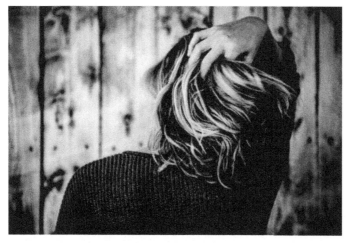

That's right – body butter has its advantages in hair care, too.

Most body butter contains coconut oil, which has numerous advantages for your hair and skin. It ensures that the body butter can protect your hair similarly as it does your skin – it restores moisture and hydrates your hair. Additionally, the antioxidants help protect it from free radicals and other elements that may damage your hair.

These healing properties aren't limited to affecting the natural elements. Using heat on your hair for beauty purposes, such as blow-drying or straightening your hair, also causes significant damage that body butter can help treat.

Furthermore, rubbing body butter into your scalp can help prevent hair loss by strengthening your hair follicles. If that is not tempting enough, it can reduce dryness and itchiness, which not only makes you more comfortable but also means you won't accidentally pull out your hair, scratching your scalp for relief.

Finally, if you're someone who struggles with curly hair, body butter is a solution. Applying body butter to your hair essentially adds a little grease and moisture, making combing your hair much easier.

When applying body butter to your hair, it is essential to remember that you shouldn't simply slather it on. Instead, take a little in your hand and let your body heat melt it. Once that happens, massage it into your hair or scalp as needed. Let it rest for a while, and wash it out with warm water and shampoo (unless you're using it to tame your curls).

Remember not to put in too much. The creaminess of body butter means that adding even a little too much can make your hair too greasy.

Other uses of body butter include:

- As a makeup remover
- As a way to soften your cuticles when you get a manicure
- To treat cracked feet and moisturize and soften your feet
- To treat chapped, sore lips

If you're ready to get started with your own homemade and organic body butter, you're in the right place. One of the biggest challenges people face when they start thinking about making their personal care products is the worry that it is too difficult, especially if they don't have prior experience.

If this is a concern you share, don't worry. Making your body butter is much easier than you think. This book will guide you through everything you need to know - from the main ingredients you'll be working with, how to whip your butter, and what essential oils you should choose - as well as recipes to use as you start on your body butter journey.

Once you master the basic recipes, there are more advanced options you can try your hand at or experiment on your own. We have selected recipes designed to target specific needs, including recipes explicitly face-friendly.

Lastly, we'll explain how to preserve your homemade body butter so they last for as long as possible and explore the best ways to use your body butter. By the time you've finished reading this book, you'll be a pro at making your body butter and will be raring to experiment with your own recipes. Who knows, you may even decide to move past making products for your own personal use and explore setting up a small business from the comfort of your own home.

In the next chapter, we'll explore some of the main ingredients you'll be dealing with when making your body butter. It will ensure you have a solid understanding of the basics of body butter before you get to make them.

Chapter 2: Explaining Main Ingredients

Natural and organic body butter usually consists of simple ingredients that help retain the skin's moisture. Its name suggests that body butter is composed of natural ingredients derived from butters like shea butter, cocoa butter, mango butter, and essential oils. Each type of butter has plenty of health benefits to keep the skin hydrated and give it a natural glow. The advantage of body butter is that it contains no oil content, so no added preservatives, making it the perfect beauty product to make at home. This chapter mentions the main ingredients in natural and organic body butter and how you can incorporate them in a simple body butter recipe.

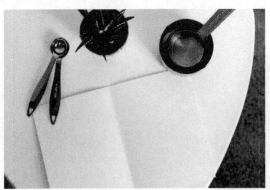

Shea Butter

Shea butter comes from the nuts of shea trees and is a common ingredient used in skincare and haircare beauty products. Due to its high vitamin and fatty acid content, shea butter has the perfect consistency for body butter and provides a soothing and hydrating effect on the skin.

Benefits

One of the key reasons it is used in many products is that it suits all skin types because its low protein content is not known to cause allergic reactions. It does not contain chemicals that may cause skin irritations. When you apply shea butter to your skin, it is quickly absorbed because its high-fat content binds with the lipid structure in the outer layers of your skin and acts as a seal to prevent moisture from escaping. The natural balance between linoleic and oleic acids in shea butter helps to give your skin a smooth texture without being too greasy.

Shea butter is also known for its anti-inflammatory, antioxidant, antifungal, and antibacterial properties, making it perfect for soothing skin irritations when exposed to dry weather. It is also rich in vitamins A and E that have anti-aging properties that fight off free radicals, one of the main factors for damaged skin cells. Triterpenes are another essential content in shea butter that has anti-aging properties as it helps delay the degeneration of natural collagen in your skin.

Studies suggest that shea butter can also help minimize the incidence of acne caused by bacteria. Shea butter has another mode of action to reduce acne. It clears out excess oil accumulated in the skin, restoring its natural oil balance. It also helps cure fungal infections that cause skin conditions like athlete's foot. Many additional health benefits gained from shea butter include healing the skin from scars faster and soothing sunburn and insect bites.

How to Buy Pure Shea Butter

When buying shea butter, specific signs will tell you whether or not it is pure, unrefined butter. Its color should be off-white, ivory white, or even close to yellow, but never bright white. A bright, white-colored shea butter tells you that it is refined and stripped of its natural nutrients, even if no additives are present. The highly refined shea butter reduces its beneficial properties present only in the purest form.

Pure shea butter should not be greasy or oily, or too hard in texture. The high levels of vitamin E in unrefined shea butter give it a firm texture, but it should melt when rubbed between your hands. It should be absorbed quickly on your skin without leaving any greasy residue.

To incorporate shea butter in a body butter recipe, you simply add it with your oil of choice, like coconut or sweet almond oil, in a heat-resistant container and place it over a water bath. This indirect heat action will cause the ingredients to melt together, and then you leave it to cool in the fridge to harden before whipping it with a hand mixer for a softer texture.

Cocoa Butter

Cocoa butter is extracted from the cocoa bean found in cocoa trees. The cocoa beans are enclosed in cocoa pods, and each pod contains around 30 seeds that are dried and squeezed to extract the natural fats that make up the cocoa butter. It is rich in fatty acids, just like shea butter, and is used in many skin moisturizers.

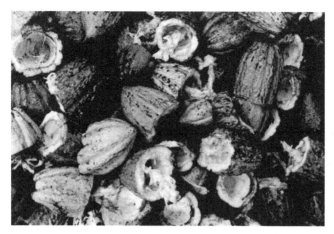

Benefits

Cocoa butter is rich in antioxidants that help prevent the damage caused by free radicals resulting from sun exposure, smoking, and other unhealthy habits. Free radicals make the skin look dull with dark patches and cause premature aging. Cocoa butter also has anti-inflammatory effects that help to give your skin a healthy glow. They may also aid in improving the appearance of scars and stretch marks on the skin as they promote faster healing.

Its high-fat content makes it ideal for body butter as it provides the skin with hydrating effects. Cocoa butter is also commonly used in lip balms because it deeply moisturizes dry and chapped skin and helps retain its moisture. It also helps heal skin irritations from conditions like eczema and dermatitis.

How to Buy Pure Cocoa Butter

Cocoa butter is available in both refined and unrefined forms. The refined form loses some of its natural nutrients, so it is best to buy the raw form of cocoa butter. It is solid at room temperature and is usually sold in bulk chunks with a pale yellow color, which resembles the appearance of soap or white chocolate. Pure cocoa butter has a distinctive strong chocolate smell, and its texture is thick in the beginning but melts as you rub it between your fingers. Refined cocoa butter is whiter and smells faintly of chocolate, unlike the raw form, and manufacturers favor refined cocoa butter because they can add different scents.

Cocoa butter can be combined with shea butter in a body butter recipe. They are melted together over a water bath or in a saucepan on low heat until incorporated together. Other essential oils and fragrances may be added, but this simple recipe will suffice as an excellent moisturizer.

Mango Butter

Mango butter is made by cold-pressing the contents of mango seeds until they form a creamy texture. It solidifies at room temperature in semi-solid chunks that resemble a waxy, almost crumbly texture and is the softest among the three butter types.

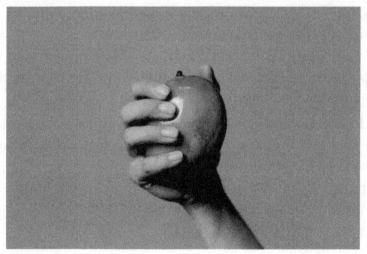

Benefits

Mango butter is a good source of antioxidants from vitamins A and E, which help minimize the damage from free radicals. It also has anti-aging effects and minimizes the breakdown of collagen fiber in the skin. Mango butter is rich in vitamin C, which increases collagen production that contributes to a healthy skin glow.

Mango butter has excellent moisturizing properties, making it a standard base for body butter. It forms a seal on the skin's surface, preventing moisture from escaping and healing chapped skin in rough areas like the heels and elbows. The high vitamin content helps protect the skin from dry weather, sun damage, and air pollutants, and some studies suggest that mango butter can even protect the skin from blue light that radiates from electronic screens.

There are no chemical irritants in mango butter, so it is safe to apply on all skin types. However, it is best not to use mango butter on your acne because of its high oil content, which can clog skin pores and worsen the condition. Use shea butter instead in this case as it does not clog the pores.

Mango butter has sunscreen effects due to its salicylic acid content, which provides skin protection from rough weather conditions when combined with vitamins C and E. It also has antimicrobial and antibacterial properties similar to shea butter that help prevent the growth of bacteria.

How to Pick Pure Mango Butter

Unrefined raw mango butter has a slightly sweet scent, unlike you might expect. It does not have a strong fruity smell because the butter is derived from mango seeds. The purest form is yellowish in color, unlike the refined butter that appears as white chunks that are more flexible and spreadable. Unrefined mango butter does not need to be heated between your fingers to produce a creamy texture. Its texture is consistent whether you take some out of the jar or if you rub it for a few seconds. Refined mango butter is a bit firmer than the unrefined type and requires a little heat from the rubbing action between your fingers to give you a creamy texture. Mango butter is refined by bleaching, and its scent is usually removed to allow other added fragrances to be more prominent.

To incorporate mango butter in a body butter recipe, follow the same process as the shea and cocoa butter. Heat it over direct or indirect heat and add your preferred fragrances and essential oils.

Coconut Oil

Coconut oil is one of the most common ingredients in skincare products. It is extracted from coconut kernels and cold-pressed until it forms coconut oil. The refined form of coconut oil is made from dried coconut meat, also known as the dry method. The other method uses pressed fresh meat to produce coconut milk and oil. The oil is separated from the milk by a fermentation process using enzymes and a special centrifuge. The pressing methods are divided into two types: hot and cold. The hot method entails pressing the coconut meat using heat or steam, while the cold method does not use heat, and it is believed that cold-pressed coconut oil retains all its beneficial nutrients.

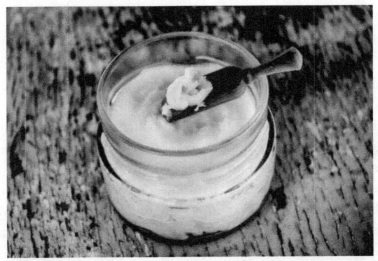

Benefits

Coconut oil contains numerous benefits to the skin as it is an excellent moisturizer and skin softener. It helps to soothe chapped skin, and its light texture leaves no residue when applied, making it suitable to apply to your skin any time during the day, and you will instantly get a softer feel on your skin.

Another valuable quality of coconut oil is that it acts as an exfoliating agent, which helps to remove dead cells from the skin. Dead skin cells make your skin seem duller and increase dark patches, leading to an older appearance. As you apply coconut oil on your skin, it eliminates sebum or excess oils in your pores, similar to the effect of shea butter, so it is an excellent ingredient to add to body butter, particularly for acne-prone skin. Its antibacterial properties help kill the bacteria on your skin that causes skin acne. This is attributed to the lauric, caprylic, and capric acid content that help fight pathogens from your skin and prevent blemishes. It will also hydrate your skin thoroughly and give it a healthy glow.

Coconut oil also has anti-inflammatory properties and soothes skin burns, inflammation, and redness from a rash or infection. It promotes skin healing and helps prevent scarring from wounds. It also contains antifungal properties, and it prevents the growth of harmful spores that cause serious skin infections, from yeast infections to ringworm.

Coconut oil can reduce the appearance of fine wrinkles to give you a younger look. It promotes cell regeneration and repair since it has been proven to increase the production of collagen fiber in the body. It is also rich in vitamin E, which contributes to skin rejuvenation. Coconut oil also acts as a deep cleanser to the skin as it removes excess oils in normal skin, not only acne skin, leaving your skin feeling cleaner and fresher. It eliminates dirt and toxins in your pores after being outdoors all day and provides your skin with healthy nutrients that keep it hydrated.

It is also used as a mild sunscreen to help prevent sun damage. It may not be sufficient for prolonged sun exposure, but it is useful in preventing sunburns if you spend some time in the sun, making it a more natural and safer option. Coconut oil also helps protect your skin against cuts from shaving, and you can use it as an alternative to your shaving cream, keeps your skin smooth, and prevents ingrown hair. It can also be applied to your underarms as an exfoliant and deodorant and prevent ingrown hairs. Instead of using a bug repellent full of chemicals, coconut oil will protect your skin from insect bites.

How to Buy Pure Coconut Oil

Unrefined or raw coconut oil solidifies at room temperature and has a distinctive strong coconut scent. Raw coconut oil is most beneficial for skin care and hair care, especially if it is extracted using the cold-pressed method mentioned earlier. Refined coconut oil is more suited for cooking and is prepared from dried coconut kernels or copra. It is designed to withstand high temperatures in cooking, and its flavor and scent are removed in the refining process, making it suitable for added flavors in food.

Pure coconut oil can be added to the cooled butter base, whether shea, cocoa, or mango butter, on direct or indirect heat to make body butter.

Aloe Vera

Aloe vera is one of the most common ingredients for skin hydration and healing products. It is extracted from the aloe plant that contains a viscous gel, which has many uses for the skin.

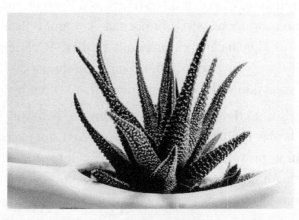

Benefits

The most widely known use for aloe vera is sunburn. It has a soothing and cooling effect on the skin with moisturizing and healing properties. Due to its aloin content, aloe vera has anti-inflammatory properties that help to reduce skin irritation, inflammation, and redness. It is also rich in metallothionein, an antioxidant protecting the skin from UV light. The soothing effect of aloe vera helps keep the skin smooth and prevents peeling after sunburn.

Aloe vera also helps to brighten the skin by giving it a natural glow. Due to excessive sun exposure and acne, the skin is susceptible to damage, leading to dark patches known as hyperpigmentation. Aloesin acts by blocking the action of melanin, which is the pigment responsible for these dark spots in the skin. Thanks to the high aloesin content in aloe vera, these dark spots can be improved.

The high water content in aloe vera gel helps retain skin moisture and prevents it from escaping. Aloe vera also contains mucopolysaccharides that increase moisture in the skin and improve the appearance of fine wrinkles as it helps maintain the skin's elastic structure. Aloe helps to increase the production of collagen, elastin, and hyaluronic acid, which all help to make the skin look younger.

Aloe also contains antimicrobial and antibacterial properties that can heal acne and is commonly used as a complementary treatment alongside acne medication. Due to its salicylic acid content, it can remove blackheads and whiteheads, one of the most stubborn skin conditions – and a tough one to get rid of. Due to its emollient properties, aloe soothes chapped and dry skin and more severe skin conditions like psoriasis. It is also thought to improve the appearance of stretch marks and scars, which is attributed to its healing properties.

How to Buy Pure Aloe Vera Gel

The color of the aloe vera gel is the first indication of whether or not it is pure and unrefined. Pure aloe vera gel is not entirely transparent or bright green. It is more of a faded yellowish or golden but translucent color, depending on its time of harvest. The pure gel must be stored in the fridge, or its color will turn brown due to oxidation.

Pure aloe vera gel does not have a fragrance, so it has been added if your product has a sweet fragrance. Another clue can be found in the list of ingredients. Ensure that your gel contains Aloe Barbadensis Leaf Extract as the main ingredient and stay away from other products containing too many items in the ingredients list.

You can easily incorporate your aloe vera gel with your base butter after melting, cooling, and mixing them into a soft texture.

This chapter listed a few ingredients that are commonly found in body butter. We discussed the benefits of each ingredient and how to use them in a body butter recipe. These ingredients are the base of body butter, so use them to get started with your recipes.

Chapter 3: Main Butter Whipping Techniques

Body butter is made using whipping techniques to ensure the end product is a creamy product you can easily spread on your skin. A creamy texture is also useful to make the body butter easily absorbed by your skin. There are two main whipping techniques in making homemade body butter; both are discussed in this chapter.

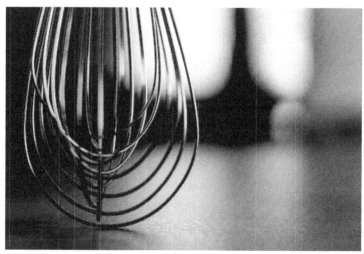

How to Choose Your Ingredients for Whipped Body Butters

Whipping techniques are used to make body butter at home. The product's texture is a bit firmer than body lotions and creams, but it is still creamy enough to give your skin a luxurious feeling with a deep moisturizing effect. The problem with making body butter is it can be a bit harder to combine, unlike lotions and creams. As discussed in the previous chapter, the base of body butter mainly consists of shea butter, cocoa butter, or mango butter. But other types can also be used, depending on the effect you want to get from a body butter recipe.

You will need to use a carrier oil or butter that is firm or solid in texture when you make your body butter. Shea butter is the ideal body butter base because it has the perfect consistency for whipping techniques. It is firm enough to produce the body butter texture, and it still easily melts between your fingers for ideal skin absorption. Other butter bases may need a bit of alteration or additives to help them reach the desired consistency of body butter.

There are different textures of each butter base. Some butter has hard textures like cocoa and kokum butter. These butter bases may be used without any additives in a body butter recipe, but do not expect them to be incredibly soft, like using shea butter. They have tremendous benefits to the skin, but the feel of the texture might be a bit firmer than you expect from a body butter. A good solution is to use a combination of hard butter with soft butter. Another substitution is to use a carrier oil to blend with a hard butter base, which will ensure a creamier texture.

While shea butter has the perfect consistency for a body butter base, there are other types of butter with a much softer consistency, including mango, murumuru, and cupuaçu butter.

These cannot be used alone in a recipe, and you will need to add another ingredient to make a firmer texture, typical of body butter. A common additive is wax or a harder butter-like illipe or cocoa butter.

Other common additives in body butter recipes that solidify at room temperature but easily melt as soon as you rub them between your fingers include coconut oil, monoi oil, and babassu oil. Since they easily melt when exposed to minimum heat, they are hardly ever used as a body butter base. They must be combined with harder butter or wax to achieve the ideal consistency of body butter. Common soft butter includes sweet almond butter, macadamia butter, olive butter, avocado butter, aloe butter, and hemp seed butter. These also require a high content of hard butter to solidify their texture enough for body butter.

Let's look at the types of waxes you can use to make whipped body butter. They help make the semi-solid texture of carrier oils and soft butter bases a lot firmer. You have to be careful with the percentage of wax used in your recipes. Adding too much wax will give you a product that is too firm, a bit like a lip balm.

Jojoba ester is a type of wax commonly used in whipped body butter recipes because it doesn't give you a waxy texture but still makes your body butter firmer. Candelilla wax can also be used, but bear in mind, it is a bit harder in texture than jojoba ester, so you can't use too much in your recipe to avoid a brittle body butter. Another common ingredient is beeswax that you can use for recipes not requiring a lot of wax because too much can give you sticky body butter.

Other additives are used to improve the body butter textures but are not used in basic recipes. More advanced recipes include ingredients that prolong a body butter's shelf-life and provide it with a specific texture. These ingredients are only to be used once you get the hang of simple recipes.

Body butter does not need preservatives due to its lack of water content, which is the main reason for the growth of bacteria and mold. However, they are still prone to oxidation and can go rancid if not stored properly, and this is why some people add antioxidants in their recipes to prevent it from happening.

Rosemary oil is a common antioxidant used in body butter, but its green color will interfere with the color of your desired product. Its fragrance may mask other additives used to produce a scent, so you may want to consider this when creating your recipe. A better option would be Vitamin E T50, an odorless and colorless antioxidant that can be used without altering the appearance and scent of your body butter.

Cornstarch is another common ingredient that helps reduce the greasy texture of body butter. The ideal ratio of cornstarch is a teaspoon for every one or two ounces of butter base. You can first blend the cornstarch with a carrier oil to avoid lumps before adding it to the base butter. An alternative to cornstarch is silk powder, which can be added at a maximum of 5% in the whole recipe. It is best to combine it with a melted carrier oil before mixing it with the rest of the ingredients.

Basic Instructions and Tips for Body Butter Recipes

When you first start with your recipes, try the one with minimal ingredients. It is the best way to get you started without feeling frustrated about not getting the right texture. Start with a small batch and use a scale to get all the measurements right. It is easier to use metric measurements when you want to increase the batch size. The batch size will indicate the type of technique used to make your body butter. There are two main whipping techniques, the cold whipping technique and the hot whipping technique, and will be discussed later in this chapter.

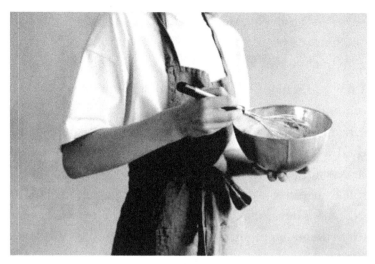

To create a basic recipe for body butter, use the few directions as follows:

1. The hot whipping technique involves tempering the base butter before use, which might be the first step in your recipe.

2. After the tempering phase, melt the base butter with the wax and carrier oil at a high temperature. This process is preferably done in a double boiler.

3. As soon as all the ingredients are melted together, remove the double boiler from the heat immediately.

4. At this stage, add any additives to enhance texture or fragrances for the desired aroma and benefits. You can leave the essential oils for the next step when the butter is cooler.

5. While the mixture is cooling, whip the ingredients together using a hand mixer for best results. Use a standing mixer if you are making a bigger batch.

6. The mixture should start to thicken as it becomes cooler. Use a spatula to scrape the sides to ensure you use every bit of the ingredients.

7. Your endpoint should be a creamy, fluffy mixture similar to cake frosting. Transfer the mixture to a sealable container, and leave to cool completely before using.

A few issues may arise during or after formulating your recipe. A common issue is that some butter may undergo crystallization. This happens when they solidify at room temperature and are exposed to heat several times for melting. You can accidentally cause crystallization because you had to melt the butter a couple of times since it can solidify while preparing or weighing other ingredients. They could also crystallize in their packages before you purchased them due to the storage conditions they were exposed to.

The tiny crystals that form on the surface of the butter change their consistency to a grainy texture. They cause no harm to your skin since they will usually melt as you rub them between your fingers or on your skin, but nobody wants grainy body butter on their skin. The whole idea of body butter is to leave your skin feeling smooth and silky, so a gritty texture won't be ideal. If you have a butter base that crystallizes for any reason, the best solution is to temper them to break down any crystals.

To temper a base butter, place it in a double boiler, a heat-resistant container on top of a pot filled with water, and place it on medium-low heat. A microwave won't dissolve the crystals, so the double boiler is more effective. When the butter starts to melt, raise the heat gradually for half an hour to 45 minutes until the butter is melted completely. The next step is to immediately stir the melted butter to eliminate any crystals left from melting. The melted butter must be transferred to a jar to cool immediately and placed in the fridge to prevent crystal formations.

Alternatively, use an ice tray to pour your mixture in before you place it in the fridge to allow it to cool quicker. Once cooled, store them in a plastic container in a cool, dark place until you are ready to use them in your recipe. Bear in mind, if they melt for any reason, they will recrystallize, and you will have to temper them once again. Whipped butter usually melts in hot weather, so don't make a big batch during summer because melting will constantly change its texture. It is one of the main reasons many people choose only to make body butter during the cooler seasons.

Remember, all the basic instructions and tips provided above serve as guidelines for your basic body butter recipe. Feel free to experiment with your recipes once you get the hang of the simple ones outlined in this book. We encourage you to keep all the tips mentioned above in mind for the best results.

Melt + Whip Technique

This technique involves tempering the butter, as discussed previously. The basic idea is to melt all your butter together in a double boiler and add all the additives. Allow them to cool in the fridge to achieve a semi-solid consistency before whipping them in a standard mixer or a hand mixer to achieve a fluffy, creamy body butter texture. This texture is perfect for allowing rapid skin absorption without clogging your pores. The concept is to create a protective seal for your skin to prevent moisture escaping, ideally without leaving a greasy residue.

The hot whipping technique is excellent for making a small batch. Let's say you are only making a one-pound worth of product. This makes the whole process of melting the butter, cooling, and finally whipping it manageable. You can get the whole thing done in under two hours maximum. But, if you want to make a five-pound batch or more, the process can be a lot harder to manage. You will have to deal with transferring hot butter into smaller containers and emptying a big chunk of your fridge space to cool them. So, the process becomes a bit of a hassle in large batches.

Here's a basic recipe using the hot whipping method:

1. Use a heat-resistant glass bowl as the top of a double boiler on a saucepan over medium heat.

2. Place a quarter cup of shea butter and mango butter each (or cocoa butter) in the glass bowl and melt completely.

3. Add one and a half teaspoons of arrowroot (flour starch or cornstarch as alternatives) to a quarter cup of carrier oil (like coconut or monoi oil). Only use the carrier oil if you don't want to use arrowroot to enhance the texture.

4. Once the butter is melted, remove the double boiler from the heat, add the carrier oil, and stir until combined.

5. Transfer the mixture to another bowl and place it in the fridge for between 30 minutes and an hour until the mixture turns into a semi-solid consistency.

6. Add 36 drops of essential oil of your choice, depending on the desired effect. For example, you can use lavender oil and sandalwood oil for a calming effect or peppermint and grapefruit oils for an energizing mixture.

7. If you choose cocoa butter instead of mango butter, make sure the mixture is whipped well using a hand mixer.

8. Place the mixture in a sealable jar and store it at room temperature in a dark, cool place.

When using body butter, it is essential always to wash your hands to prevent bacteria growth. This body butter recipe can last for about six months with proper use. Massage a small amount on your skin after a shower. If you use mango butter, your end product will be softer and creamier as it is a softer butter. You can also use cocoa butter for that delicious chocolate smell, but the texture of your body butter will be a lot firmer than if you used mango or shea butter. Consider using the arrowroot to eliminate the possibility of a greasy texture.

Cold Whip Technique

The cold whipping technique is much easier and faster because it requires fewer steps. Let's take shea butter as an example base butter:

1. Cut the bigger pieces into smaller pieces and place them in a bowl for mixing.

2. You can use a hand mixer at high speed or a standard mixer for larger batches.

3. Make sure you scrape off the sides to combine all the butter pieces.

4. Once the butter is broken down, add all your additives from carrier oils to essential oils while continuously mixing until you reach a fluffy consistency.

5. Transfer your body butter to containers for later use.

6. Make sure you store in a dark, cool place to avoid melting. The cold whipping technique takes a lot less time so that you can create a ten-pound batch in under an hour.

This method can only be used with softer butter bases like shea butter, cupuaçu butter, and mango butter because they are easily whipped without using heat. While the harvesting season may affect their firmness, they can still be cut into smaller pieces for cold whipping. Other harder butter, like cocoa butter and waxes, has a harder texture, and you must use the hot whipping method.

There are a few advantages to the cold whipping method over the hot method. Whipping the ingredients without melting gives you a better indication of what the end product feels like. With the hot technique, you will get a fluffier texture that will turn firmer when left to cool and set, so you won't be able to alter the texture after the mixture is cooled completely. You can better control the texture in the cold method because you end up with a texture you can use immediately after formulation.

Essential oils lose some of their health benefits when heated, which is why you have to wait for the butter to cool down in the hot method before adding them. This gives the cold method an advantage because you can add the essential oils, carrier oils, and any other additives at any time during whipping. The cold method does not entail excess equipment like the hot technique, which requires a double boiler and other containers for cooling.

Here's a simple recipe using the cold whipping technique:

1. Place half a cup of shea butter in a bowl. It is best to use shea butter at room temperature for easier whipping. You can either cut the shea butter into chunks or use a fork to make it smaller.

2. Add two teaspoons of jojoba oil to the mixture.

3. Whip the mixture for about two minutes at high speed.

4. Add the essential oils while whipping for an extra minute to incorporate all ingredients.

5. The end product should be a creamy mixture similar to cake frosting.

6. Place the mixture in a piping bag using a spatula, as it is easier to fill your smaller containers for later use. You can use a plastic bag as an alternative by gathering the mixture in a corner and cutting a small part of the tip.

This simple recipe can be used as whipped body butter, and the formulation serves as the base for many recipes to experiment with. You can use different essential oils for different effects. For example, add a few drops of Frankincense to turn the mixture into a moisturizing eye cream. The possibilities are endless with this basic recipe.

This chapter discussed how to use different ingredients to make whipped body butter. We mentioned the differences between the hot and cold whipping techniques and when to use them. Use this information to guide the process of executing the recipes and to create your own body butter recipes.

Chapter 4: Choosing Essential Oils

When making your skincare products, there are many ingredients you need to consider. Essential oils are an extremely, if not the most important part of any skincare product. In addition to imparting amazing fragrances to your products, they also help deal with skin problems. Every essential oil has distinctive properties, but each one ultimately makes your skin soft and supple. Body butter is a favorite for many of us, but without essential oils, they'd lose half their charm. This chapter will dive deep into the different properties of essential oils and explain how they benefit the skin to help you better understand the purpose of essential oils in body butter formulations.

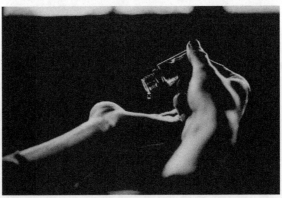

Why Add Essential Oils?

Do you ever wonder why essential oils are so essential for skincare products? Well, not only are they used for aromatherapy, but they also provide fantastic skin-loving properties. For example, tea tree oil is an excellent antiseptic. Similarly, peppermint oil increases circulation, whereas lavender contains a naturally soothing fragrance. These oils are added to skincare products to make them unique, scent-wise, and property-wise. Body butter is mainly used to nourish dry skin, but combine it with the beneficial essential oils properties, and you're transforming a plain butter and oil mixture into a unique product with its own specific properties.

How Much Should You Add?

Essential oils are highly concentrated, and therefore you should be cautious when adding them to skincare products. Did you know that it takes 60 whole roses to make just 1 drop of rose essential oil? Let that settle in, and then re-evaluate the amount you use in your products. Adding too much makes your product excessively fragrant and also harmful to your skin. Never use essential oils liberally on your skin, and definitely don't ingest them.

It is recommended that you use around 1-2% essential oils in your body butter mixes. For a 1% ratio, 6 drops of essential oils should be added to every 1 oz. of oil and butter. For a 2% ratio, add 12 drops of essential oils to 1 oz. of oil or butter.

Top Essential Oils for Body Butter

Your choice of essential oils depends on the skin benefits you're seeking and the scent you prefer. Each essential oil has its properties and provides numerous benefits to your skin. Listed below are the top essential oils you can use when making body butter.

1. Lavender

Lavender essential oil has a unique aroma and countless exceptional properties resulting in its numerous uses everywhere. From treating stress and fatigue to nourishing dry skin and rough patches, lavender essential oil is a go-to option for many. It is one of the most utilized essential oils for homemade skincare products.

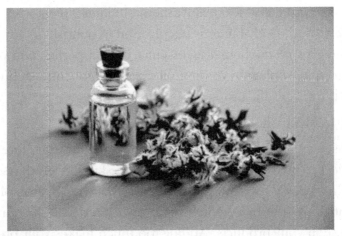

Properties

- Lavender is famous for relieving stress, anxiety, fatigue, and depression.

- Its scent relieves feelings of nausea and sickness and eases headaches.

- Lavender essential oil, helps improve sleep and relaxes your mind and body.

- It can help alleviate menstrual cramping.

- Lavender essential oils are famous for their antibacterial properties.

Skin Benefits

- Lavender is packed with antioxidants to protect your skin and nourish it.

- The antibacterial properties of lavender help treat acne flare-ups.

- Its anti-inflammatory properties reduce inflammation and skin irritation.

Possible Side Effects

- Some individuals may be allergic to lavender essential oil and may experience skin irritation or nausea. If so, discontinue use immediately.

- If you are nursing or pregnant, consult your doctor before use.

2. Chamomile

Chamomile oil is directly extracted from the flowers of its plant. It has been considered a medicinal herb for centuries, and there are a surprising number of health benefits for using chamomile essential oil.

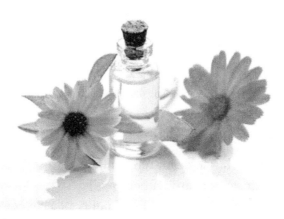

Properties

- Chamomile has extremely beneficial antibacterial and antiseptic properties.

- It has incredible antidepressant qualities that help relieve anxiety and depression.

- Its scent is said to relax your mind and help you sleep better.

- Chamomile oil has analgesic properties that relieve pain in muscles and joints.

- It can help alleviate menstrual cramping.

Skin Benefits

- Due to its anti-inflammatory properties, it soothes your skin complexion and reduces acne, irritation, and rough skin patches.

- The antioxidants in chamomile essential oil flush out toxins and improve circulation, resulting in reduced acne, hyperpigmentation, and blemishes.

Possible Side Effects

- Skin irritation can be observed after using concentrated essential oils or products containing them. Before use, test the product or oil on a small patch of skin to ensure you're not allergic.

- If you're taking prescription medication, chamomile oil could interact with them and cause problems.

- If you are nursing or pregnant, consult your doctor before use.

3. Clary Sage

Clary sage oil has a clean, refreshing scent used extensively in skincare products and aromatherapy. There's a lot of scientific evidence claiming the numerous benefits of clary sage essential oil for your skin and otherwise.

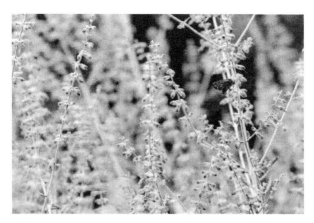

Properties

- The scent of clary sage essential oil helps alleviate stress by inducing a state of well-being in your mind.

- Its antibacterial properties ensure no toxins or bacteria accumulate on your skin.

- Considered a natural antidepressant, it helps reduce feelings of stress and sadness.

- It can help alleviate menstrual cramping

Skin Benefits

- Clary sage has stimulating properties that trigger circulation, detoxify your skin, and rejuvenate your complexion.

- Clary sage oil contains an ester that reduces skin inflammation and soothes skin.

- Clary sage essential oil is famous for balancing your hormones and regulating sebum secretion to reduce breakouts, acne, and oily skin.

Possible Side Effects

- For people with low blood pressure, using clary sage essential oil is not recommended.

- If you are nursing or pregnant, consult your doctor before use.

4. Sandalwood

Sandalwood essential oils are used in many perfumes and skincare products because of their classic scent. But the use of sandalwood essential oil goes far beyond its smell. It has numerous skin and health benefits, making it a perfect choice for skincare products, especially body butter and the like.

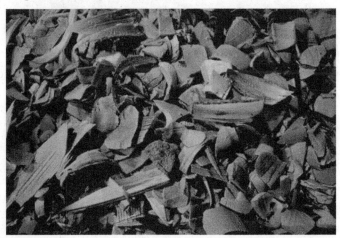

Properties

- Sandalwood essential oil promotes mental clarity and improves cognitive function, resulting in a stress-free state of mind.

- Sandalwood is used to speed up tissue and muscle repair and helps nourish damaged skin.

- It further acts as an antiseptic and protects your skin from future infections.

- Its scent creates feelings of peace and calm and helps reduce problems associated with anxiety and depression.

Skin Benefits

- Sandalwood essential oil can help replenish dry skin by penetrating your skin layers deeply and hydrating it.

- It has an amazing anti-aging effect, as it gently tones and tightens the skin around wrinkles.

- It soothes the epidermis layer of your skin and moisturizes and nourishes your skin.

Possible Side Effects

- If you are nursing or pregnant, consult your doctor before use.

5. Rosemary

Rosemary essential oils have been used for years in skincare products, and people especially prefer to use them in homemade products. It has a woody aroma and numerous health and skin benefits.

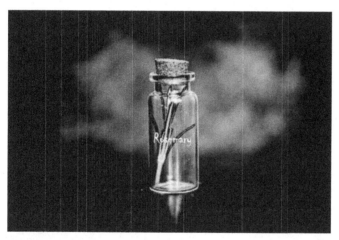

Properties

- Rosemary essential oil is famous for a brain and nerve tonic and improving cognitive function. It can treat depression, anxiety, and forgetfulness.

- It is used to control the cortisol levels of your brain and hence helps reduce chronic stress tremendously.

- It improves blood circulation and helps you feel rejuvenated.

- With its stimulating properties, it can help alleviate menstrual cramping.

Skin Benefits

- Rosemary oil consists of antibacterial elements that help cleanse your complexion and leave your skin feeling refreshed.

- It helps balance the regulation of natural oils in your skin and ensures your skin is nourished.

Possible Side Effects

- Some individuals may be allergic to rosemary and experience skin irritation or nausea. If so, discontinue use immediately.

- If you are nursing or pregnant, consult your doctor before use.

6. Geranium

Geranium oil is widely used as an ingredient in perfumes, cosmetics, and self-care products. Due to its many properties, it is used in skin care and aromatherapy for numerous health benefits.

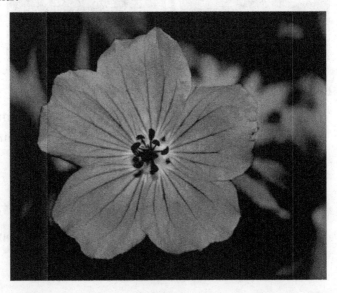

Properties

- Geranium oil is said to rebalance your nervous system and boost your mood. It provides your brain with a feel-good element that helps reduce stress, anxiety, and depression.

- It has anti-inflammatory and antibacterial properties that significantly fight against many issues.

Skin Benefits

- Geranium oil acts as an astringent and an anti-aging agent. It tones and protects your skin and also reduces fine lines and wrinkles.

- It has anti-inflammatory properties that help purify and soothe your skin and smooth out your complexion.

- It rejuvenates your skin by controlling sebum production.

Possible Side Effects

- Allergic reactions are possible - test before using geranium oil in your products.

- If you are nursing or pregnant, consult your doctor before use.

7. Neroli

Neroli or orange blossom essential oil has a citrus, fruity scent and is mainly used to provide fragrance to products. Due to its soothing effect, it is used in skin-care products like lotions, balms, and body butter.

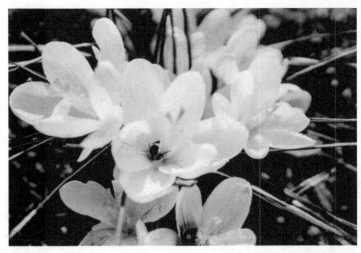

Properties

● Due to its calming effects, orange blossom essential oil improves your sleep.

● Its powerful scent can relieve feelings of anxiety, depression, and fatigue.

● Neroli essential oil helps improve sleep and relaxes your mind and body.

Skin Benefits

● Neroli oil intensely moisturizes your skin and boosts cell generation in the epidermis layer.

● Its antibacterial properties are used to target breakouts and help regulate sebum production.

● Whether you have dry or oily skin, sebum regulation, when controlled with Neroli oil, can help get the perfect oil balance.

● It hydrates, revives, and purifies your skin by penetrating deep into the epidermis layer.

Possible Side Effects

- Some individuals may be allergic to Neroli essential oil and experience skin irritation or nausea. If so, discontinue use immediately.

8. Tea Tree

Tea tree oil has many properties, including antibacterial to skin-loving qualities. It is mainly used in natural skincare remedies for preventing fungal infections and healing damaged skin.

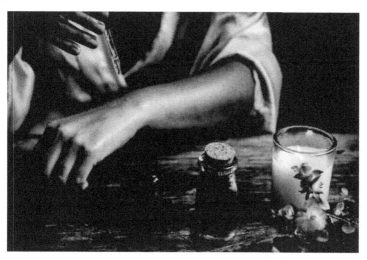

Properties

- Its antibacterial properties help treat bacterial infections and prevent future infections.

- Tea tree essential oil has commendable stimulating properties that enhance circulation and improve your overall health and well-being.

- Its scent can relieve feelings of nausea and sickness and ease headaches.

Skin Benefits

- It helps purify your skin by removing toxins and hence prevents acne and breakouts.

- Equipped with anti-inflammatory properties, it calms your skin and soothes any irritation.

- It repairs, strengthens, and protects the epidermis layer in your skin.

Possible Side Effects

- Although tea tree oil is safe for most people, it may cause irritation and swelling.

- For people with acne, tea tree oil could trigger severe allergic reactions.

9. Lemon

Lemon essential oils are widely used as a natural ingredient in many homemade skincare products. It has numerous skin benefits that promote healthier and fresher skin.

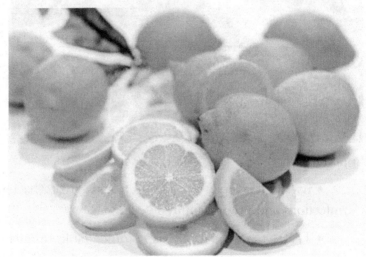

Properties

- Lemon essential oil is a natural solution to help ease feelings of nausea and vomiting.

- Due to its antimicrobial properties, it has an amazing purifying effect on your body.

- Its scent and soothing effect can help relieve stress, anxiety, depression, and fatigue and make you feel relaxed.

Skin Benefits

- Lemon essential oil is rich in antioxidants and therefore helps energize your skin.

- It has strong hydrating properties that help rejuvenate your skin and repair damaged or dried skin by penetrating the epidermis layer.

- It restores your skin's natural oil balance and manages sebum production.

Possible Side Effects

- Lemon essential oil is highly concentrated and can be sensitive to the skin. Some individuals may be allergic to it and notice undesirable skin reactions as a result.

10. Cistus

Cistus essential oil is present in diluted and absolute forms and is used in the formulation of cosmetics and fragrances due to its unique scent and amazing skin-loving properties. It has calming and grounding properties and, when added to products, can soothe and relax your mind and body.

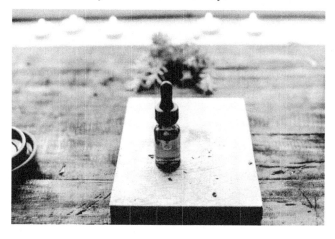

Properties

• Due to its antiseptic and antibacterial properties, cistus essential oil is widely used to purify and cleanse.

• Its anti-inflammatory properties can help soothe tender and damaged skin.

• It aids your respiratory system and helps improve sleep, and relaxes your mind and body.

Skin Benefits

• Cistus oil is exceptionally soothing for the skin. It can help treat sunburns, acne, hyperpigmentation, and even acne spots. This oil penetrates deep into the epidermis layer to calm the afflicted area.

• It can reduce fine lines and wrinkles around tight spots of your skin and rejuvenate it.

• It helps heal broken and damaged epidermis layers and remove scars.

Possible Side Effects

• Cistus oil is not recommended for young children.

• If you are nursing, pregnant, epileptic, have liver damage, or have other medical problems, consult your doctor before use.

11. Peppermint

Peppermint oil is known for its sharp, fresh odor that provides a refreshing experience for the user. It is used in many cosmetics and skincare products to improve skin texture and provide a cool, fresh look.

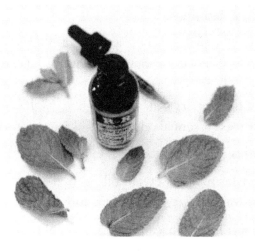

Properties

- Its soothing scent can help suppress feelings of nausea and reduce headaches.

- It helps relieve muscle and joint pain and reduces inflammation.

Skin Benefits

- Peppermint oil has stimulation properties that heal and strengthen the epidermis layer by deep penetration.

- Peppermint mainly comprises methanol, a natural cooling agent, dealing with irritation, puffiness, and oily skin.

- Due to its strong antimicrobial properties, it helps combat acne and cleanses your pores resulting in smoother, clearer skin.

• Possible Side Effects

- Some individuals may be allergic to peppermint herb or essential oil and experience skin irritation or nausea. If so, discontinue use immediately.

12. Jasmine

Jasmine essential oil has a distinct flowery aroma and a plethora of distinct qualities, owing to its wide range of applications. It is a popular choice for alleviating stress and fatigue and healing dry skin and rough spots. It is one of the most commonly used essential oils in DIY skincare products.

Properties

- Jasmine essential oil is well-known for alleviating tension, anxiety, exhaustion, and depression.

- It has antibacterial and antiviral properties, so they're extensively used in medicines.

- It promotes restful sleep and relaxes the mind and body.

- It can help alleviate menstrual cramping, regulate hormone levels and other PMS symptoms.

- Jasmine essential oil's ingredients boost brain activity and awaken your mind.

Skin Benefits

- This essential oil is rich in antioxidants that stimulate cell regeneration and prevents premature aging.

- It provides natural rehydration and opens your pores. As a result, your skin will be nourished after use.

- Jasmine oil regenerates your skin cells, evens your skin tone, and reduces hyperpigmentation and acne scars.

Possible Side Effects

- Some individuals may be allergic to jasmine essential oil and experience skin irritation or nausea. If so, discontinue use immediately.

13. Vetiver

Vetiver essential oil has many skin and health benefits in medicinal and cosmetic formulations. It is used extensively in homemade skincare products and has an aromatic scent that attracts many.

Properties

- Vetiver has naturally soothing properties and treats nervous system disorders, mainly stress, ADHD, autism, and nervousness.

- It is a stimulant and a natural tonic that helps soothe every system of your body.

- It has antibacterial properties that prevent infections.

- It is used to relieve anxiety and depression due to its relaxing scent.

Skin Benefits

- Due to its powerful antibacterial properties, vetiver essential oil can help cleanse your skin by unclogging pores and removing pollutants and toxins.

- It promotes skin cell regeneration and heals dry and damaged skin.

- Vetiver essential oil, packed with antioxidants, rejuvenates the skin by reducing thin lines and wrinkles.

Possible Side Effects

- Ensure that you don't use this oil in a concentrated form.

- Take caution when applying to the skin as it may cause allergic reactions for some individuals.

- If you are nursing or pregnant, consult your doctor before applying to the skin or ingesting.

14. Frankincense

Frankincense is also known as the king of essential oils because of its numerous benefits and uses. With its ability to rejuvenate your mind and body, it has been used for centuries in beauty products. This essential oil is an important component for many products, from aromatherapy to medicine and cosmetic formulations.

Properties

- Frankincense oil has been proven to affect your mental health positively and is used to treat anxiety, stress, and depression problems.

- Its antiseptic properties boost your body's immunity to infections and viruses.

- Frankincense oil can regenerate tissues and skin cells due to its astringent nature and results in renewed and strengthened skin.

- Its contents can help boost cognitive function and enhance brain activity.

Skin Benefits

- Frankincense oil is packed with antioxidants that help protect your skin, rejuvenate, and nourish it.

- It helps balance the sebum production in the epidermis layer and maintains your skin's oil balance.

- Its anti-inflammatory properties help reduce inflammation and skin irritation.

Possible Side Effects

- Some individuals may be allergic to this essential oil and experience skin irritation or nausea. If so, discontinue use immediately.

- If you are nursing or pregnant, consult your doctor before use.

15. Rose

Everyone loves the smell of roses. Its essential oil has ten times the fragrance and benefits that roses bring. Rose essential oils are present in diluted and absolute forms and have many benefits.

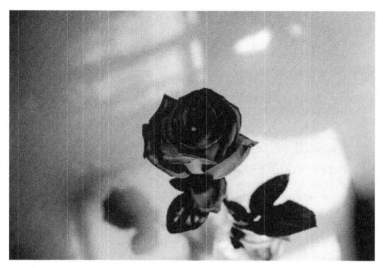

Properties

- Rose essential oil is a natural antioxidant that detoxifies and purifies your skin and promotes healthy living.

- It has strong antimicrobial properties that help prevent infections.

- Rose oil has been proven to improve your mood and confidence by inducing a feeling of well-being into your mind. Therefore, it is used to treat anxiety and depression.

- One of the most significant benefits of rose essential oil is its antispasmodic nature that can help relax and soothe your nerves and skin.

Skin Benefits

- Due to its anti-inflammatory nature, rose essential oil is an excellent addition to improving your skin's glow. It helps fight against irritation and puffiness.

- It can heal, regenerate, and protect the epidermis skin layer and is hence used as an anti-aging product.

- It makes your complexion brighter and reduces hyperpigmentation and acne scars.

Possible Side Effects

- Due to the highly concentrated solution of rose essential oil, ensure that you use a stringent amount in every product.

- Some individuals might be allergic, so it is important to test it on your skin before use.

Chapter 5: Basic Recipes to Try Now

This chapter discusses body butter recipes you can make at home. We focus on easy recipes that won't take much of your time or money. Additionally, the ingredients we mention are all organic and natural, which won't cause any allergies or skin irritation. When choosing between buying commercial brands and making body butter at home, the choice is very simple. Organic products are the better option because they lack the harsh chemicals found in their counterparts, making them gentler on the skin. People are now more conscious of what they apply to their skin, and they look for better and healthier alternatives. Your skin will absorb whatever you apply to it, so you should be careful with the products you use. Making organic products like body butter at home will give you control over what ingredients you use and what ingredients to avoid.

If you look at the list of ingredients on any commercial product, you will notice they use different chemicals, some you may have never heard of before. Even retail brands that claim all of their products are natural still use some questionable ingredients. For instance, many brands include a fragrance on their list of ingredients, but how can you guarantee they use natural scents and not synthetic ones? Synthetic fragrances aren't good for your health since they may cause allergic reactions. As a rule, you shouldn't put something on your skin if you don't feel safe putting it in your mouth.

In addition to safe ingredients, making homemade body butter is cheaper than buying commercial brands. We have dedicated this chapter to some easy and fast recipes that will help get you started and save you time and energy.

Easy Coconut Oil Body Butter Recipe

The coconut oil body butter recipe is very easy and won't take you more than twenty minutes to make. If you have cracked or dry skin, this body butter will be a great addition to your skin routine. The coconut oil will moisturize and nourish the skin, while shea butter will leave your skin feeling hydrated. Additionally, shea butter will protect your skin from the sun since it has natural SPF factors. The recipe also includes cocoa butter and sunflower oil that protects the skin from signs of aging and irritation. The essential oils will also give it a lovely scent. However, if you prefer odorless body butter, you can simply opt out of using essential oils.

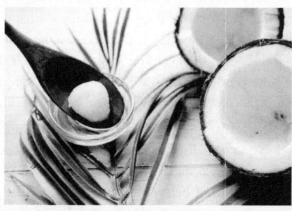

Ingredients

- Coconut Oil - 3 tbsp
- Refined Shea Butter - 2 tbsp
- Cocoa Butter - 2 tbsp
- Sunflower Oil - 4 tbsp
- Carnauba Wax - 0.5 tsp
- Ylang-Ylang Essential Oil - 3 drops
- Frankincense Essential Oil - 3 drops
- Palmarosa Essential Oil - 5 drops

Where to Find Ingredients

You can find all of the ingredients on Amazon, so all you need to do is go online and order them right away.

Directions

1. Let the shea butter, cocoa butter, carnauba wax, and coconut oil melt in a double boiler

2. When melted, add the sunflower oil

3. Next, leave in the freezer for about 15-20 minutes

4. Remove from the freezer when hardened but not frozen

5. Mix the ingredients with a hand blender until you achieve a creamy mixture

6. Now, you can add the essential oil (optional)

7. Place the body butter in a container/s

Tips and Tricks

1. Melt the ingredients on low to medium heat

2. You can add a teaspoon of Brazilian nut oil to your recipe if desired

3. Although you can substitute the sunflower oil, it may affect the product's texture

4. You can increase the amount of the cocoa butter and shea butter if you want to make the body butter more solid

Ingredient Substitutions

Coconut oil	Monoi oil
Sunflower oil	Almond oil
Carnauba wax	Beeswax (you will have to increase the quantity)

Simple Shea Body Butter Recipe

Shea body butter contains vitamins E and A, which balances and hydrate the skin. The addition of mango butter to the recipe will help regenerate the skin due to its healing qualities. The recipe also includes chamomile flower water that calms the skin. After showering, apply the shea body butter on your whole body to moisturize your dry skin. This recipe won't take over 10 minutes to prepare and make.

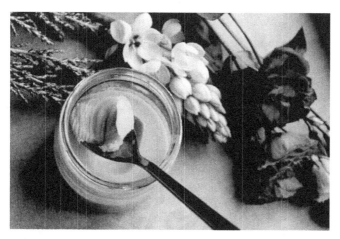

Ingredients

- Organic Shea Butter - 5 tbsp
- Organic Grapeseed Oil - 3 tbsp
- Organic Mango Butter - 2 tbsp
- Oil Phase 83%
- Water Phase 8%
- Chamomile Flower Water - 1 tbsp
- Organic Beeswax Pellets - 1 tbsp
- Lavender Essential Oil - 10 to 15 drops
- Natural Emulsifier - 8%

Where to Find Ingredients

You can find the ingredients on websites like Amazon or any market near you. You can check any organic or aromatherapy store online or near you for the oils.

Directions

1. Let the shea butter, beeswax, and oil melt in a double boiler

2. Next, add the chamomile flower water

3. When the ingredients have melted, mix them together until you achieve a creamy liquid mixture

4. Now, add the essential oil and stir thoroughly to mix with the ingredients

5. Then pour the ingredients into a glass container

6. Leave until it solidifies

Tips and Tricks
1. If the finished product is greasy, you can add arrowroot powder 2. Avoid using aloe vera gel because it may decrease the shelf life

Ingredient Substitutions	
Grapeseed oil	Jojoba oil

Fast Mango Body Butter Recipe

Mango body butter is easily absorbed by the skin, leaving it soft and smooth and moisturizes the skin the moment you apply it. Although mango butter has a very pleasant scent, it smells nothing like mangoes. Mango body butter is an excellent treatment for sensitive and dry skin. It also reduces scars, wrinkles, and stretch marks. Additionally, the body butter moisturizes and calms sun-dried skin.

Ingredients

- Organic Unrefined Mango Butter - 12 tbsp
- Roman Chamomile Essential Oil - 15 drops
- Patchouli Essential Oil - 10 drops
- Organic Safflower Oil - 6 tbsp
- Organic Refined Shea Butter - 2 tbsp
- Bergamot Essential Oil - 3 drops

Where to Find Ingredients

You can easily find all of the ingredients on Amazon and the oils at an aromatherapy store near you.

Directions

1. Fill a pan with water and let the mango and shea butter melt in a heatproof glass bowl in the pan.

2. Leave the stove on low heat for the butter to melt slowly.

3. Add the safflower oil and mix it with the melted butter.

4. Leave the glass bowl in the freezer for about 5 to 10 minutes until it becomes thick.

5. Next, set your electric whip to slow speed and whip the mixture.

6. Keep whipping until you achieve a fluffy-like texture.

7. Next, increase the whip's speed to medium.

8. When you have finished whipping, add the essential oils.

9. When your body butter looks and feels like whipped cream, it means that it is done.

Tips and Tricks

1. For smoother skin, you can add arrowroot powder

2. Use a deep bowl to avoid the butter flying around

3. Wear an apron

4. Increase the mango butter if the finished product starts melting

5. Avoid over-whipping it

Ingredient Substitutions	
Safflower essential oil	Jojoba essential oil
Bergamot essential oil	Jasmine or lavender essential oil

Whipped Body Butter

The addition of vegetable glycerin is great for people with skin irritation as it calms the skin. Additionally, the arrowroot powder will make the body butter less greasy, while essential oils give it a very pleasing scent. The whipped body butter will hydrate, nourish, and protect the skin.

Ingredients

- Organic Safflower Oil - 10 tbsp
- Vegetable Glycerin - ½ tbsp
- Arrowroot Powder - ½ tbsp
- Organic Refined Shea Butter - 7 tbsp
- Ho Wood Essential Oil - 3 drops
- Lavender Essential Oil - 5 drops
- Rosewood Essential Oil - 5 drops
- Patchouli Essential Oil - 3 drops

Where to Find Ingredients

All of these ingredients are found on Amazon. You can also find them in a market or organic store near you.

Directions

1. Fill a pan with water.

2. Add the safflower oil and shea butter to a heatproof glass bowl and put it in the pan.

3. On low heat, let them melt slowly.

4. When they have melted, mix in the arrowroot powder.

5. Next, put the mixed ingredients in the freezer for about 5 to 10 minutes until they develop a soft or wax texture.

6. Add the vegetable glycerin and essential oils.

7. Whip the mixture using an electric mixer, setting it on a low speed until it develops a creamy texture.

8. When the butter feels fluffy like whipped cream, it means it is done.

Tips and Tricks	
1. Adding the vegetable glycerin is optional 2. The mixture shouldn't be frozen, or you won't be able to whip it 3. Avoid overmixing	
Ingredient Substitutions	
Shea butter	Cocoa butter
Safflower essential oil	Sunflower essential oil

The Simplest Ucuuba Body Butter Recipe

The Ucuuba butter is a seed extracted from a plant under the same name. It has a nice scent and is a remedy for many skin conditions due to its anti-inflammatory quality. It can also restore the skin's texture and tone.

Ingredients

- Raw Ucuuba Butter - 6 tbsp
- Organic Jojoba Oil - 3 tbsp

• Organic Refined Shea Butter - 3 tbsp

Where to Find Ingredients

You can find the oils at an aromatherapy store near you, while the butter and tools can be found on Amazon or any market near you.

Directions

1. Fill a pan with water.

2. Get a heatproof glass bowl and put the shea butter and ucuuba butter in it.

3. Put the glass bowl in the pan.

4. Leave it on low heat and let the butter slowly melt.

5. Mix in the jojoba oil with the mixture.

6. Leave the mixture in the freezer for about 5 to 10 minutes until it feels soft and thick.

7. Whip the mixture with an electric whip that is set on a low speed.

8. Keep whipping until the mixture reaches a fluffy texture.

9. Increase the mixer speed until it feels creamy.

Tips and Tricks	
Hemp oil will be an excellent ingredient for people with eczema. You can use it instead of jojoba oil.	
Ingredient Substitutions	
Jojoba oil	Hemp oil

Whipped Cocoa Body Butter

Cocoa butter has an intense moisturizing quality and calms skin inflammation. It can also reduce and prevent the appearance of stretch marks. Additionally, cocoa butter is rich in antioxidants to protect and soothe the skin. Moreover, cocoa reduces any marks on your skin, including signs of aging like wrinkles and scars. The jojoba oil in the recipe will leave your skin soft and moisturized, while coconut oil will protect and repair your skin.

Ingredients

- Cocoa Butter - 10 tbsp
- Jojoba Oil - 8 tbsp
- Coconut Oil - 2 tbsp

Where to Find Ingredients

You can find the ingredients in a market near you while the oils are in an organic or aromatherapy store.

Directions

1. Put all of the ingredients in a glass container.

2. Make sure it is heatproof.

3. Let the ingredients melt in a double boiler.

4. Set the heat on low.

5. Make sure that you stir the ingredients while they are melting.

6. Wait until the ingredients melt before you remove them from the heat.

7. Cover the bowl and leave it in the fridge for an hour.

8. Remove them from the fridge once they feel cool and soft.

9. Get an electric blender and use it to blend the mixture for a few minutes.

10. Stop blending once the mixture reaches the desired texture.

11. Your coca body butter is all done now, so put it in a container and start using it.

Tips and Tricks	
If you want a strong scent, you can opt for raw cocoa butter, but if you want a softer scent, opt for refined cocoa butter.	
Ingredient Substitutions	
Coconut oil	Apricot oil
Jojoba oil	Almond oil

Easy Argan Oil Body Butter

Argan oil nourishes the skin, keeps it soft, and protects it from various elements. Argan oil is also very beneficial for oily skin since it regulates oil production.

Ingredients

- Argan Oil - 1 tbsp
- Shea Butter - ¼ cup
- Coconut Oil- ½ cup
- Cornstarch - 1 tbsp
- Geranium Essential Oil - 7 drops
- Lavender Essential Oil - 7 drops

Where to Find the Ingredients

You can find the ingredients in a market or an organic store near you. The ingredients are also available on Amazon.

Directions

1. Melt the shea butter in a double boiler and set on medium-low heat
2. Wait until the shea butter is soft
3. Next, put it in a glass container
4. Add argan oil and coconut oil to the shea butter
5. Whip the ingredients for about 3 minutes
6. After whipping, add the cornstarch to the mixture
7. Beat the mixture again for 5 minutes
8. Once the mixture develops a creamy texture, put it in a glass jar

Tips and Tricks
This body butter can also be used as a shaving cream or as a remedy for cracked heels

Ingredient Substitutions	
Shea butter	Cocoa butter
Coconut oil	Almond oil

Honey Body Butter Recipe

The combination of honey, shea butter, and cocoa butter will hydrate and repair your skin. The chamomile essential oil will soothe and nourish the skin while giving it a refreshing scent. Additionally, the body butter will leave your skin radiant, supple, and moisturized. The cocoa butter will also give it a chocolate-like fragrance.

Ingredients

- Honey - 1 tbsp
- Shea Butter - 3.5 tbsp
- Cocoa Butter - 25 grams
- Sweet Almond Oil - 35 grams
- Chamomile Essential Oil - 10 drops

Where to Find Ingredients

You can find the ingredients in any market or aromatherapy store near you.

Directions

1. Put the cocoa butter and shea butter in a saucepan.

2.   Get another pan and fill it with water.

3.   Put the saucepan in the pan with water or use a double boiler.

4.   Let the butter melt.

5.   After it melts, take the saucepan, and put it on a potholder.

6.   Next, add the honey and sweet almond oil.

7.   If the oils start solidifying, put the saucepan in the water pan again.

8.   Wait until the oils melt.

9.   Pour the ingredients into a glass container.

10.   Put it in the freezer for about 5 minutes.

11.   Take the glass container out to add and mix the essential oils with the mixture.

12.   Put it back in the freezer for 5 to 10 minutes.

13.   Take the container out of the freezer and whisk the mixture one last time.

Tips and Tricks	
If you don't want to use cocoa butter, you can just add extra shea butter.	
Ingredient Substitutions	
Sweet almond oil	Olive oil
Shea butter	Coconut oil

Chamomile Body Butter Recipe

Chamomile is known for its soothing quality, and it can heal damaged skin. The addition of beeswax will allow the skin to absorb moisture, while coconut oil will hydrate and cleanse the skin. If you want to feel energized, you can add essential oils to the ingredients.

Ingredients

- Dried Chamomile Flower - 2 tbsp
- Coconut Oil - ¼ cup
- Shea Butter - ½ cup
- Sweet Almond Oil - 2 tbsp
- Jojoba Oil - 2 tbsp
- Beeswax - 1 ½ tbsp
- Bergamot Essential Oil - 10 to 20 drops

Where to Find Ingredients

You can find the ingredients on Amazon or an organic store. If you find it hard to find any of the ingredients, you can search online for stores that sell soap ingredients. You will find online stores or markets near you that sell them.

Directions

- Put the shea butter, jojoba oil, coconut oil, sweet almond oil, wax, and chamomile flowers together in a bowl.
- Place the bowl with the ingredients in a double boiler and stir them together.
- Set the heat to just over medium.
- Let the ingredients melt.
- Next, remove the bowl from the double boiler.
- Remove the flowers strain.

- After the ingredients cool down, put the bowl in the fridge until it begins to solidify.

- Then whip the ingredients for about 3 to 5 minutes.

- You will notice the mixture starts to develop a fluffy texture.

- Place it in a glass jar and start using your new homemade body butter.

Tips and Tricks	
If you don't have chamomile flowers or tea, you can make the body butter without it. The recipe will still work.	
Ingredient Substitutions	
Beeswax	Organic sunflower wax/organic soy
Dried Chamomile flowers	Chamomile tea
Bergamot essential oil	Lavender/ylang-ylang essential oil

Vanilla Body Butter Recipe

The vanilla body butter has a very delightful fragrance. The addition of aloe vera gel will help hydrate and calm the skin since it contains many antioxidants, while coconut oil and shea butter will nourish and hydrate the skin.

Ingredients

- Vanilla Extract - 1 ½ tbsp
- Coconut Oil - ½ cup
- Shea Butter - ½ cup

- Aloe Vera Gel - 1 tbsp
- Vitamin E Oil - 1 tbsp
- Beeswax Pastilles - 2 tbsp
- Mica Powder- 1 dash

Where to Find Ingredients

You can find the ingredients on Amazon or in a market or organic store near you.

Directions

1. Prepare a double boiler.

2. Put the beeswax, coconut oil, and shea butter in the double boiler and let them melt.

3. Stir the ingredients while they are melting.

4. After the ingredients melt, remove them from the double boiler.

5. Leave for 10 minutes to cool down.

6. Next, add the vanilla extract, aloe vera gel, and the mica powder to the mixture.

7. Use a blender or a mixer to whip them together.

8. Keep whipping until the body butter develops a soft texture.

9. Place the mixture in a container.

10. Leave it overnight to cool down.

Tips and Tricks
1. Using aloe vera gel from a plant is better than a bottle since it is more natural. 2. 1 tbsp of aloe vera gel = 6 small aloe vera leaves.
Ingredient Substitutions

Coconut oil	Any carrier oil you want
Shea butter	Any type of butter
Vanilla extract	Essential oil

All of the recipes mentioned in this chapter are very easy and won't take more than 20 minutes to make. They are all made with natural ingredients that will not hurt your skin or cause any allergies. Once you master these basic ingredients, you can start making more complicated ones.

Chapter 6: Complicated but Yummy Recipes

After experimenting with your basic recipes, it is time to try out a few advanced ones. While the whipping techniques might be the same with all the recipes, a few extra steps make a recipe much better. We encourage you to try out the advanced recipes outlined in this chapter to explore different types of body butter that give you more beneficial effects on your skin.

Body butter formulations can be a bit tricky when you are attempting to achieve the correct consistency. One of the main issues with texture is the grittiness and greasiness of the base butter. The previous chapters already established how shea butter is a popular butter base in body butter formulations because it provides the best consistency. It is the reason many formulators will use shea butter in almost every body butter recipe. They combine it with other butter to create different formulas. We discussed some basic recipes to get you acquainted with the process. Now, let's take a look at a few complicated recipes to try.

Coconut Ginger Body Butter

This moisturizing body butter gives a warming sensation due to the added spices. It has a delicious gingerbread smell, making it perfect for the holiday season. All you need is to apply it after your shower, grab a cup of hot cocoa, and watch your favorite movie while tucked under a cozy blanket.

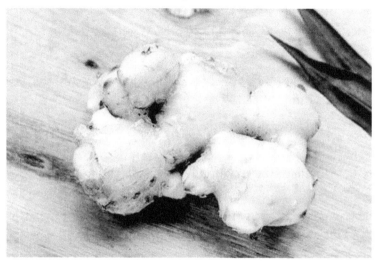

Ingredients

- Coconut Oil - ½ cup
- Shea Butter - ½ cup
- Vanilla Extract - 2 tsp
- Ground Ginger - 2 tsp
- Cinnamon - 1 tsp

Where to Find Ingredients

You can find all these items on Amazon, makingcosmetics.com, or any other website specializing in wholesale cosmetics products. You can find the spices at your local grocery store.

Directions

1. Place the coconut oil with the shea butter in a saucepan over low heat.

2. Once the shea butter is melted, whisk the ingredients well until incorporated.

3. Take the saucepan off the heat and allow it to cool down to room temperature.

4. Place the mixture in a bowl and place it in the fridge for 20 minutes.

5. Take the bowl out of the fridge and add the rest of the additives.

6. Use a hand mixer to whip the mixture for three minutes.

7. Place the mixture in a sealable jar.

8. Store in a dark, cool place for six months.

Tips and Tricks
1. If you make a bigger batch, use a standard mixer for easier whipping.   2. Make sure your fingers are clean each time you use the body butter to prevent bacteria growth and make it last longer.   3. The body butter may separate in storage. Simply stir the mixture with a whisk or a spatula until incorporated.

Ingredient Substitutions	
Coconut oil	Sweet almond oil
Cinnamon powder	Nutmeg powder

Mango Citrus Body Butter

This rejuvenating body butter is the perfect way to start your day. It has a rich mango and citrus scent you will look forward to every time you wake up in the morning. This body butter is perfect for applying right after your morning shower without having to reapply during the day. It will act as the perfect seal for your skin, preventing moisture from escaping from its outermost surface.

Ingredients

- Shea Butter - ½ cup
- Coconut Oil - ½ cup
- Mango Butter - ½ cup
- Almond Oil - 1 cup
- Citrus Essential Oil - 30 drops

Where to Find Ingredients

You can find all the items on Amazon, makingcosmetics.com, or any other website specializing in wholesale cosmetics products.

Directions

1. Place the mango butter, shea butter, and coconut oil in a heat-resistant bowl over a pot filled with water over medium heat.

2. Once all the butter is melted together, add the almond oil and citrus oil, and mix well.

3. Allow the mixture to cool down to room temperature.

4. Place the bowl in the fridge for an hour.

5. After one hour, take the bowl out of the fridge and blend the mixture using a hand mixer until a smooth, fluffy mixture is formed.

6. Transfer the contents to a sealable jar.

7. Store in a cool, dark place for up to six months.

Tips and Tricks

1.   If you want to create a relaxing body butter for nighttime, replace the citrus oil with lavender or chamomile oil.

2.   You can also create a body butter suitable for rejuvenation during the afternoon by replacing the citrus oil with peppermint oil.

3.   Try replacing your essential oils each time you create this recipe until you find the right combination for you.

Ingredient Substitutions

Coconut oil	Sweet almond oil or babassu oil
Mango butter	Murumuru butter or cupuaçu butter
Almond oil	Olive oil

Vanilla Bean Body Butter

This body butter is made a bit differently than other body butter. The main base is not a nut butter type but a natural unscented lotion. It is combined with cocoa butter to improve its gritty texture and make it smoother. The lotion base makes the body butter more hydrating and moisturizing to the skin. Its warm fragrance notes provide a calming effect due to its high essential oil content.

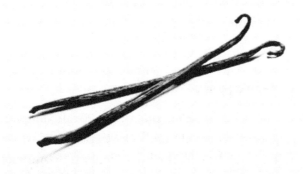

Ingredients

- Natural Unscented Lotion - 200 ml
- Cocoa Butter -100 g
- Vanilla Bean Oil - 10 drops
- Benzoin Oil - 1 ml
- Clove Bud Oil - 4 drops
- Jojoba Rose Oil - 1 ml
- Evening Primrose Oil - 30 ml

Where to Find Ingredients

You can find all the items on Amazon, makingcosmetics.com, or any other website specializing in wholesale cosmetics products.

Directions

1. Place the cocoa butter in a heat-resistant bowl over a pot filled with hot water over medium heat.

2. Allow the cocoa butter to melt until it reaches a liquid state.

3. Place the unscented natural lotion base in a bowl.

4. Use a hand mixer to whisk the lotion base as you gradually pour in the liquefied cocoa butter.

5. When the cocoa butter is incorporated with the lotion base completely, add the evening primrose oil while continuously whisking the mixture with the hand blender.

6. Continue mixing until the lotion and oil are combined with no visible separation.

7. Add the benzoin oil, vanilla bean oil, sandalwood oil, jojoba rose oil, and clove bud oil while mixing continuously until all the ingredients are combined.

8. Cover the bowl with plastic wrap and allow it to cool down in a cool, dark place until it sets.

9. The end product is a creamier version of whipped body butter.

10. Place the contents in a sealable jar and store it in a cool, dark place for six months.

Tips and Tricks	
1. Use a standard mixer for easier pouring of the essential oils to allow a steady mix and prevent separation of the ingredients.	
Ingredient Substitutions	
Vanilla oil	Sandalwood oil or myrrh oil
Clove bud oil	Cinnamon oil, lemon oil, or oregano oil

Mango Turmeric Body Butter

This body butter is a bit trickier to produce because of the yellow stain of turmeric oil. Turmeric is known to brighten the skin and improve the appearance of scars because it promotes cell regeneration and healing. It is what makes it great for eliminating dark spots from prolonged exposure to sunlight.

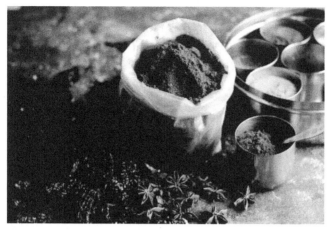

Turmeric contains anti-inflammatory effects, making it suitable for skin conditions like acne, eczema, and psoriasis. Another great benefit of turmeric is its anti-aging properties because it promotes collagen fiber production and delays its degeneration in the body. It also contributes to the wound healing effect. The apricot oil content in this recipe helps the body butter to be rapidly absorbed by the skin without leaving any greasy residue.

Ingredients

For the turmeric infusion:

- Turmeric Powder - 3 tbsp
- Jojoba Oil - 180 ml
- Vitamin E - 15 drops

For the body butter recipe:

- Shea Butter - 137.5 g
- Mango Butter - 50 g
- Apricot Kernel Oil - 20 g
- Turmeric Infused Oil - 37.5 g
- Pumpkin Spice Oil - 1.25 g

• Arrowroot Powder - 3.75 g

Where to Find Ingredients

You can find all the items on Amazon, makingcosmetics.com, or any other website specializing in wholesale cosmetics products.

Directions

To make the turmeric-infused oil:

1. Use empty tea bags to add the turmeric powder and tie them with the attached string.

2. Add the jojoba oil to a glass container and place the tea bags inside.

3. Fill the rest of the jar with jojoba oil and close it tightly.

4. Place the jar in a pot filled with water on low heat for 3 hours.

5. Make sure to check the mixture every hour or so to replace the evaporated water.

6. Remove the jar from the heat and allow it to cool down to room temperature.

7. Add the vitamin E oil, stir well until combined, and store in a cool, dry place.

To make the body butter recipe:

1. Place the shea butter and mango butter in a double boiler until melted.

2. Add all the liquid oils, stir, and heat for two extra minutes.

3. Remove the mixture from the heat, transfer to another bowl, and continue stirring with a spatula. This technique is used to prevent the grittiness of shea butter.

4. Once the mixture has cooled down, add the arrowroot powder, and mix until fully incorporated.

5. You can add essential oils or fragrances at this stage.

6. Continue stirring as the mixture becomes viscous until the spatula leaves traces in the bowl. You can place it in a larger bowl filled with ice-cold water to make the mixture cool faster.

7. Place the bowl in the fridge for 30 minutes to solidify.

8. Take the mixture out of the fridge and whip it using a hand mixer.

9. Place the contents in a sealable jar.

10. Store in a cool, dark place for six months.

Tips and Tricks
1.   Depending on your preference, you can experiment with different essential oils in this recipe, like ginger oil, vanilla bean oil, sandalwood oil, or pumpkin spice oil. 2.   Only use turmeric powder to create your infusion. If you use turmeric root, you may not get rid of all the moisture, allowing bacterial growth causing the body butter to become rancid. 3.   You can substitute the jojoba oil in the turmeric oil infusion with sweet almond oil, sunflower oil, rice bran oil, or soybean oil.

Ingredient Substitutions	
Apricot kernel oil	Safflower oil, rosehip oil, or grapeseed oil

Arrowroot powder	Tapioca starch, flour starch, or cornstarch

Honey Body Butter

This thick body butter is deeply moisturizing for your skin. You can use it after your shower for a luxurious feeling and leave you with a natural glow. The comfrey-infused sweet almond oil promotes skin healing, but pregnant women or children should avoid it. If you are pregnant, use sweet almond oil as the carrier oil in this recipe without performing the comfrey leaves infusion step.

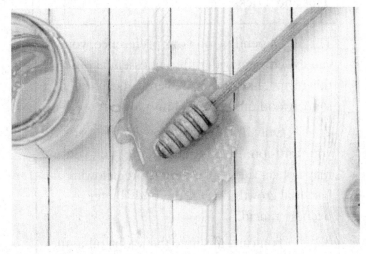

Ingredients

For the comfrey infusion:

- Sweet Almond Oil - 473 ml
- Dried Comfrey Leaves - 2 cups

For the body butter recipe:

- Honey - 7 g
- Cocoa Butter - 25 g
- Shea Butter - 50 g

- Comfrey-Infused Sweet Almond Oil - 35 g
- Chamomile Essential Oil - 10 drops

Where to Find Ingredients

You can find all the items on Amazon, makingcosmetics.com, or any other website specializing in wholesale cosmetics products. Make sure to buy organic raw honey free from beeswax, or you can filter it out to ensure a smooth consistency for your body butter.

Directions

To make the comfrey-infused sweet almond oil:

1. Place the leaves in a sealable jar until it reaches about two-thirds of the surface. You can tear the leaves to make them fit better inside the jar.

2. Pour the sweet almond oil into the jar until it is filled to the top.

3. Wait to see if the leaves absorb the oil making the oil level go down.

4. Pour some more oil until the jar is filled.

5. Store the jar at room temperature in a dark place for 4 to 6 weeks.

6. Shake the jar every day to ensure proper infusion.

7. After 4 to 6 weeks, strain the oil using a strainer lined with cheesecloth to remove the leaves.

8. Store in a dark place for up to a year.

To make the body butter recipe:

1. Place the shea and cocoa butter in a saucepan on top of a pot filled with water over medium heat.

2. Remove the saucepan as soon as the butter is melted.

3. Add the honey and infused sweet almond oil and blend using a whisk.

4. If you see any chunk residues from the butter, place the saucepan back on the heat.

5. Place the saucepan in the freezer for about five minutes.

6. Add the essential oil, mix, and freeze for five more minutes.

7. A thin layer should form on the surface of the mixture. Whisk the mixture once more.

8. Immediately pour the contents into a jar because the ingredients will solidify quickly.

9. This body butter can be used for up to six months if stored correctly.

Tips and Tricks
1.   Ensure that the comfrey leaves are completely dried before infusing them with sweet almond oil. Any moisture will allow bacterial growth, which will shorten its shelf-life. 2.   Purchase organic raw honey without any beeswax residue to ensure a smooth body butter texture.

Ingredient Substitutions	
Cocoa butter	Kokum butter or illipe butter
Shea butter	Mango butter
Chamomile oil	Lavender oil, lemongrass oil, or carrot seed oil

Avocado Infusion Body Butter

This body butter provides a deep moisturizing effect to your skin, leaving it silky and smooth. The avocado oil is infused with cinnamon, cardamom, and cloves to induce a warming sensation on your skin, making you feel more relaxed. This body butter is perfect for use right before going to bed to promote a good night's sleep. Avocado oil acts as an emollient that moisturizes dry skin and helps heal rough areas in the skin like the elbows and heels. This recipe also includes babassu oil, which is packed with antioxidants and fatty acids that contain antibacterial and antimicrobial properties suitable for acne-prone skin.

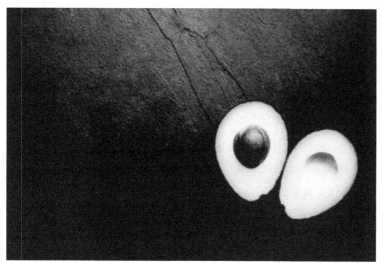

Ingredients

For the avocado infusion:

- Avocado Oil - 100 g
- Cardamom - 1.5 g
- Cinnamon - 2.2 g
- Cloves - 2.2 g

For the body butter recipe:

- Shea Butter - 130 g

- Cocoa Butter - 10 g

- Babassu Oil - 27.5 g

- Avocado Infusion - 67 g

- Hypericum Extract (Also called St. John's Wort) in Sunflower Oil - 12.5 g

- Tocopherol - 2.5 g

- Ginger Essential Oil - 0.5 g

Where to Find Ingredients

You can find all the items on Amazon, makingcosmetics.com, or any other website specializing in wholesale cosmetics products. You can get the spices at your local grocery store or spice shop. Make sure you ask for the unrefined shea and cocoa butter to gain the most benefits from each. Organic butter is less greasy and has a better texture than refined butter.

Directions

For the avocado infusion:

1. Place the cinnamon, cloves, and cardamom in a mill and crush them until finely ground.

2. Add the ground spices to the avocado oil and mix them well until you get a homogenous mixture. The result should be a dark green oil.

3. Let the mixture stand for about 30 minutes.

4. Filter the mixture to obtain the infused avocado oil leaving the spices behind. The spices did their part and are discarded to avoid a grainy texture for the body butter.

For the body butter recipe:

1. Place the babassu oil with the shea butter and cocoa butter in a heat-resistant container.

2. Place the container in a pot filled with water on medium heat to create a double boiler.

3. Allow the butter to melt and incorporate with the oil.

4. Once the butter is melted, take the container off the heat.

5. Add the avocado oil, St. John's Wort extract, and tocopherol, and stir gently.

6. Continue stirring until the mixture cools down to about 35C and add the ginger essential oil.

To make a conventional body butter:

1. Place the above mixture in a jar, or you can continue blending in the current container until the mixture cools down to room temperature.

2. Continue stirring until the mixture becomes more viscous to the point where your spatula leaves a trace.

3. Place the mixture in a jar and put it in the fridge for cooling for 12 hours up to 24 hours. This method helps to prevent the base butter from crystallizing.

4. The end product is a smooth, firm body butter without a grainy texture.

To make a whipped body butter:

1. Repeat the above steps until you reach the consistency when your spatula leaves traces in your container.

2. Use a hand mixer to whip your mixture until you reach a cake frosting consistency. You should be left with a smoother, fluffier texture than the conventional method.

3. Place in the fridge for 12 hours up to 24 hours. Let it come down to room temperature before use.

4. The end product is a paler shade of green with a fluffy, smooth texture.

Tips and Tricks	
1. Make sure to use organic and refined avocado oil for best results. 2. Pure shea butter is off-white or slightly yellowish and not bright white. 3. Pure cocoa butter has a pale-yellow color, resembling raw white chocolate chunks. It also has a distinctive strong chocolate smell, unlike the refined kind.	
Ingredient Substitutions	
Cocoa butter	Kokum butter
Ginger oil	Lavender oil
Babassu oil	Coconut oil

This chapter outlined a few recipes you can try once you master basic formulas. With advanced formulations, you can substitute different ingredients to create various body butter that provides a wide range of effects. We hope the information provided in this chapter serves as a guide for your explorations and experiments with organic ingredients to make your body butter recipes.

Chapter 7: Body Butter for Specific Purposes

You'd be surprised to know that body butter is used for purposes other than moisturizing your skin. Although they're mainly used for moisturizing, body butter is designed to treat many other problems. Whether it is to treat dry knees and elbows or moisturize your hair, the versatility of these products is so broad, and they can be used for numerous things.

Unlike standard self-care products, homemade body butter is free of harsh chemicals that can damage your skin and cause severe allergic responses. Homemade body butter contains natural components that help heal dry skin, rashes, irritation, and dead skin.

This chapter outlines how to create different body butter to deal with specific problems. The recipes are pretty straightforward and designed for special needs while addressing the significant moisturizing solution.

All Body Moisturizing Whipped Body Butter

As mentioned previously, body butter is mainly used to moisturize your skin and leave it feeling soft and hydrated. Specific body butter is designed to be more moisturizing than others to treat very dry skin, especially in winter. One of these is the all-body moisturizing whipped body butter. Combined with whipped coconut oil and aromatic essential oils, this body butter takes care of all your moisturizing needs as it can be applied to any part of your body. Although it is a little greasy, it blends perfectly to nourish and hydrate the epidermis layer when applied to your skin.

Ingredients

- Coconut Oil - ⅓ cup or 76g
- Shea Butter - ⅓ cup or 76g
- Jojoba Oil - ⅓ cup or 76g
- Cocoa Butter Wafers - ⅓ cup or 76g
- Arrowroot Powder - 2 tbsp or 30g
- Essential Oils - As desired

Where to Find Ingredients

Coconut oil, Jojoba oil, and essential oils can be found at any cosmetic or skincare market. Shea butter and Cocoa butter wafers can be found in any grocery store near you. Arrowroot powder can be found online or in the spice section of a grocery store.

Directions

1. Melt the cocoa butter, shea butter, and coconut oil in a double boiler or microwave over low heat.

2. When melted, remove the mixture from heat and add Jojoba oil to the mix.

3. Create an essential oil blend according to your preferences and incorporate it into the body butter mixture.

4. Pour the mixture into a large bowl and refrigerate until solidified (for about 2 hours).

5. After the mixture solidifies, place it at room temperature and whip it with either a hand or an automatic mixer until it is light and airy.

6. While whipping the solution, add arrowroot powder and keep mixing.

7. Finally, scoop out the mixture and pour it into a glass jar. Store in a cool, dry place.

Tips and Tricks
1.   You can use the following essential oil blend for a fresh fragrance: • Peppermint (15 to 20 drops)   • Frankincense and Lavender (15 drops each)   • Grapefruit and lime (20 drops each)   • Vanilla and Lavender (15 drops each)   2.   Ensure that you store the body butter in a cool place. Otherwise, the mixture will start to melt and lose its properties.

Ingredient Substitutions	
Jojoba oil	Sweet almond oil/ fractionated coconut oil/ olive oil.
Coconut oil	Mango Butter

Body Butter for Hair Revitalization

This DIY recipe is specially designed for nourishing dry and damaged hair and contains shea butter to hydrate the tips and roots of your hair. If you want an easy hair revitalizing solution, this body butter should be your go-to recipe. It contains all-natural nourishing ingredients and a lavender scent to top it off.

Ingredients

- Shea Butter - 1 cup or 227g
- Jojoba Oil - 2 tbsp or 28g
- Avocado Oil - 2 tbsp or 28g
- Rosehip Oil - 2 tbsp or 28g
- Olive Oil - ¼ cup or 57g
- Lavender Oil - 10 drops

Where to Find Ingredients

Jojoba oil, Olive oil, Avocado oil, Rosehip oil, and essential oils can be found at any cosmetic or skincare market. Shea butter can be found in any grocery store near you or online.

Directions

1. Heat the shea butter, jojoba oil, avocado oil, and rosehip oil in a double boiler for two hours.

2. Pour the melted mixture into a bowl and wait for it to start solidifying at room temperature.

3. Add the lavender essential oil to the mix and use a mixer to whip the solution.

4. As you mix it, gradually add the olive oil, and keep whipping it until it is a frothy, light batter.

5. Finally, scoop out the mixture and pour it into a glass jar. Store in a cool, dry place.

Tips and Tricks	
1. Make sure you add a suitable amount of olive oil when whipping the mixture, as it will ensure the final product is in a lathery, foamy state and not solidified or lumpy. 2. Ensure that you store the body butter in a cool place. Otherwise, the mixture will start to melt and lose its properties.	
Ingredient Substitutions	
Jojoba oil	Sweet almond oil/ fractionated coconut oil/ olive oil.
Lavender oil	Any other essential oil of your choice.

Shea Body Butter Makeup Remover

Numerous products are present in the cosmetics industry aimed solely at makeup removal. Many of these products have harmful chemicals and are pretty expensive. This **DIY** body butter makeup remover recipe contains shea butter and coconut oil to remove all traces of makeup, dirt, and oil from your skin.

Ingredients

- Virgin Coconut Oil - ⅓ cup or 76g
- Unrefined Shea Butter - ⅓ cup or 76g
- Jojoba Oil - ⅓ cup or 76g
- Vanilla Essential Oil - 10 drops

Where to Find Ingredients

Coconut oil, Jojoba oil, and essential oils can be found at any cosmetic or skincare market. Shea butter can be found in any grocery store near you.

Directions

1. Melt the shea butter and coconut oil in a double boiler or microwave for about an hour.

2. When melted, let it cool at room temperature.

3. After the mixture cools down into a solid form, add the jojoba oil into the mix and whip.

4. While mixing the solution, add drops of vanilla essential oil for a sweet scent.

5. You can use a hand or automatic mixer to whip the mixture until a light and frothy mixture is obtained.

6. Finally, remove the mixture from the bowl and put it into an airtight jar or container.

Tips and Tricks	
1. If you have sensitive skin, replace the vanilla essential oil with any other essential oil blend. 2. Ensure that you store the body butter in a cool place. Otherwise, the mixture will start to melt and lose its properties.	
Ingredient Substitutions	
Jojoba oil	Sweet almond oil/ fractionated coconut oil/ olive oil.
Coconut oil	Mango butter

Vanilla Essential oil	Lavender/Chamomile essential oil

Anti-Itch Whipped Body Butter

Eczema causes irritation, itchiness, and rashes that can leave scars if not treated properly. Coconut oil, when combined with shea butter, is the best natural remedy for treating eczema-prone skin. This anti-itch body butter recipe has certain antimicrobial and anti-inflammatory properties that effectively target eczema spots and help minimize their appearance.

Ingredients

- Virgin Coconut Oil - 5 tbsp or 70g
- Unrefined Shea Butter - 3 tbsp or 42g
- Calendula Oil - 1 tbsp or 14g
- Castor Oil - ½ tbsp or 7g
- Vitamin E - 4 Capsules
- Lavender Essential Oil - 15 drops
- Tea Tree Essential Oil - 7 drops

Where to Find Ingredients

The oils can be found at cosmetic or skincare shops. Shea butter can be found in any grocery store near you. You'll find the vitamin E capsules at a pharmacy and online.

Directions

1. Put the unrefined shea butter, coconut oil, and castor oil in a double boiler or microwave and melt them, stirring until melted.

2. Once melted, pour the mixture into a glass bowl, and let it cool down for an hour. You can also refrigerate the solution to cool it down in less time.

3. Whip the solution with a hand mixer or a stand mixer and gradually add drops of calendula oil, lavender oil, and tea tree oil. Keep mixing while you add these.

4. Add the vitamin E oil from the capsules and whip the solution until a frothy mixture is obtained.

5. Store the mixture in an airtight container in a cool, dry place.

Tips and Tricks
1.   Make sure you do a patch test to ensure no allergic reactions occur. 2.   If you have tree nut allergies, it is important to avoid shea butter. 3.   Ensure that you store the body butter in a cool place. Otherwise, the mixture will start to melt and lose its properties.

Ingredient Substitutions	
Coconut oil	Mango butter
Lavender essential oil	Any other essential oil blend

Elbow and Knee Moisturizer

Certain spots on our body are dryer than others because of their texture. Elbows and knees are two of these and require extra attention and care to ensure they're not dry white patches of skin. This DIY recipe includes shea butter, almond oil, and many moisturizing and nourishing essential oils that ensure maximum hydration, even for dry spots like your knees and elbows.

Ingredients

- Shea Butter - ½ cup or 96g

- Isopropyl Myristate - 1 tbsp or 15g

- Sweet Almond Oil ⅓ cup or 36g

- Vitamin E Oil - 1 tsp or 0.75g

- Neroli Essential Oil - ½ tsp or 0.5g

- Grapefruit Essential Oil - 10 drops

- Rose Absolute Essential Oil - 15 drops

Where to Find Ingredients

The essential oils can be found at any cosmetic or skincare market. Shea butter can be found in any grocery store near you.

Directions

1. Place the shea butter in a glass bowl and use a hand or stand mixer to whisk it.

2. Keep whisking it until the butter gets light and fluffy (about 2-5 minutes).

3. Add the isopropyl myristate and use the mixer to blend the solution again.

4. Add the sweet almond oil, vitamin E oil, and essential oils one by one while continuously mixing the solution.

5. You should get a foam-like butter mixture at the end of the process. If not, check your measurements and try again.

6. Put into a sterile, airtight container and keep in a cool place.

Tips and Tricks	
1. Make sure you don't overdo the butter. Otherwise, the mixture will turn hard instead of soft, foamy cream. 2. Ensure that you store the body butter in a cool place. Otherwise, the mixture will start to melt and lose its properties.	
Ingredient Substitutions	
Jojoba oil	Sweet almond oil/ fractionated coconut oil/ olive oil.
Coconut oil	Mango butter
Essential oil	Any suitable blend.

Anti-Ageing Whipped Body Butter

There are tons of anti-aging creams and lotions present in the market these days. But imagine how great it would be if all your moisturizing and anti-aging needs were covered by a single product and a homemade one free of harmful chemicals and artificial ingredients. This anti-aging whipped body butter will ensure your skin remains moisturized while also reducing tightness and fine lines on your skin.

Ingredients

- Coconut Oil - ¼ cup or 57g
- Shea butter - ½ cup or 113g
- Argan Oil - 1 tbsp or 14g
- Sweet Almond Oil - 2 tbsp or 28g
- White beeswax pellets - 1 tsp or 4g

- Vitamin E Oil - 1 tsp or 4g

- Jojoba Oil - 1 tbsp or 14g

- Arrowroot Powder - 1 tbsp or 14g

- Essential Oils - As desired

Where to Find Ingredients

Coconut oil, Jojoba oil, and essential oils can be found at any cosmetic or skincare market. Shea butter can be found in any grocery store near you. Arrowroot powder can be found online or in the spice section of a grocery store. Beeswax pellets can be found in an online retail store.

Directions

1. Place the coconut oil, shea butter, jojoba oil, argan oil, sweet almond oil, and beeswax into a heatproof bowl and heat for about two hours.

2. When melted, take the solution off the heat, and let it cool down at room temperature.

3. When the solution starts solidifying, use a hand mixer to whip it until it becomes fluffy and creamy.

4. Now, place it in the fridge for about 15 minutes, then whip it again.

5. Add the arrowroot powder, essential oil blend, and vitamin E oil while gradually whipping the mixture.

6. Let the mixture form a frothy, foamy shape and shift it to an airtight container.

7. Store in a cool and dry place.

Tips and Tricks	
1. It is important that you don't overheat the oils. Otherwise, their efficacy will be significantly reduced.	
2. Add the essential oil blend after the mixture has cooled down, or the scent will fade.	
3. Ensure that you store the body butter in a cool place. Otherwise, the mixture will start to melt and lose its properties.	
Ingredient Substitutions	
Jojoba oil	Sweet almond oil/ fractionated coconut oil/ olive oil.
Coconut oil	Mango butter
Essential oil - Lavender/Chamomile	Vanilla/Tea tree oil

Cuticle Hydration

It is common to have dry and broken cuticles, especially during winter. In addition to making your fingers look unpleasant, they also hurt. This DIY cuticle hydration body butter recipe is perfect for treating rough, dry, or overgrown cuticles. This body butter is perfect for winter as it is filled with moisturizing natural ingredients, including shea butter and beneficial essential oils.

Ingredients

- Shea Butter - ¼ cup or 57g
- Jojoba Oil - 1 tbsp or 14g
- Coconut Oil - 2 tbsp or 28g

- Vitamin E Oil - 1 tbsp or 14g

- Geranium Essential Oil - 15 drops

- Rosemary Essential Oil - 15 drops

- Lavender Essential Oil - 15 drops

Where to Find Ingredients

Coconut oil, Jojoba oil, Olive oil, Avocado oil, Rosehip oil, and essential oils can be found at any cosmetic or skincare market. Shea butter can be found in any grocery store near you or online.

Directions

1. Put the coconut oil and shea butter in a bowl and microwave for 30 seconds, stir, and microwave again for 30 seconds. Ensure they're melted completely.

2. Add 1 tbsp of Jojoba and Vitamin E oil and stir to ensure uniform mixing.

3. Blend the three essential oils in a separate container, then add this blend into the mixture.

4. Let the solution cool off in small containers.

5. Ensure that your containers are airtight and store them in a cool place where the mixture won't melt.

Tips and Tricks	
Ensure that you store the body butter in a cool place. Otherwise, the mixture will melt.	
Ingredient Substitutions	
Jojoba oil	Sweet almond oil/ fractionated coconut oil/ olive oil.
Lavender oil	Any other essential oil of your choice.
Shea butter	Mango butter

Reduce Stretch Mark and Scars

Cellulite and scars are prevalent for many people. Whether it is due to pregnancy or weight changes, cellulite is a typical sight for many. While many people look for creams and chemicals to remove these marks, they ignore the side effects of these products. On the other hand, this all-natural anti-cellulite body butter does not have any hidden side effects, is affordable, and in addition to reducing cellulite and scars, it will keep your skin moisturized. The most important ingredient of this body butter is the grapefruit essential oil, which reduces cellulite and scars.

Ingredients

- Coconut Oil - ⅛ cup or 16g
- Cocoa Butter - ¼ cup or 32g
- Sweet Almond Oil - ⅛ cup or 16g
- Grapefruit Essential Oil - 15 ml

Where to Find Ingredients

Coconut oil, Almond oil, and essential oils can be found at any cosmetic or skincare market or online. Shea butter and Cocoa butter wafers can be found in any grocery store near you.

Directions

1. Melt the cocoa butter, almond oil, and coconut oil in a double boiler or microwave over low heat.

2. Put it in the refrigerator for 20 minutes, don't leave it longer, or it will harden too much.

3. When the mixture has solidified, gradually add the grapefruit essential oil while mixing.

4. Whisk the mixture using a hand or stand mixer until a foamy, creamy mixture is obtained.

5. Spoon out the mixture into an airtight jar or container and keep it in a cool place.

Tips and Tricks

1.   You can use the following essential oil blend for a fresh fragrance:

- •   Peppermint (15 to 20 drops)
- •   Frankincense and Lavender (15 drops each)
- •   Grapefruit and lime (20 drops each)
- •   Vanilla and Lavender (15 drops each)

2.   Ensure that you store the body butter in a cool place. Otherwise, the mixture will start to melt and lose its properties.

Ingredient Substitutions

Cocoa butter	Shea butter
Almond oil	Coconut oil

Chapter 8: Body Butters for Your Face

Body butter is excellent for moisturizing and hydrating your skin. The body butter consisting of shea butter is fabulous on your face as it consists of omega-3 fatty acids. It is essential to use butter that is non-comedogenic in your body butter so that it won't clog your pores. You must consider the ingredients present in the product when using it on your face.

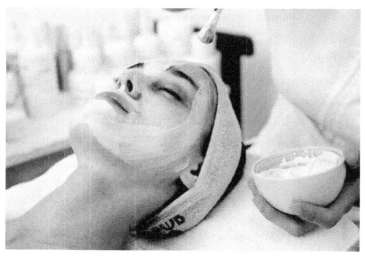

Is Body Butter Safe to Be Used on Skin?

Body butter is an excellent moisturizer. It hydrates your skin and nourishes it to look and feel smoother and softer. Moreover, it is important to know that the skin on your face is different from the rest of your body. Your facial skin contains more oil glands and is thinner than other areas of your body. It does not mean that your face will have a bad reaction to body butter. However, if you have oily or acne-prone skin, it may not be a good choice to use body butter on your face. If you have normal skin, you can safely use body butter on your face as a moisturizer, or if your skin is oily, use ingredients that are not greasy.

The store-bought body butter may cause itchiness or redness on your skin because it could contain an allergen ingredient. So, make your DIY body butter using safe ingredients for your skin. This chapter discusses a few DIY body butter recipes safe to use on your face. Most of these recipes are safe for sensitive skin, but you must check the ingredients to see if they contain irritants.

Whipped Body Butter with Shea Butter

The whipped body butter with shea butter is an excellent choice if you're looking for a moisturizer suitable for your face. This body butter is very light as the recipe consists of beating the mixture in intervals to create tiny air pockets, making it extremely soft and smooth on the skin. The whipped body butter can be used daily as it nourishes and softens your skin with vitamins to keep it healthy and smooth. The variety of essential oils like Neroli and sweet almond oil give it the sweet scent that makes it even more pleasant to use.

Ingredients

- Shea Butter - 97 g
- Sweet Almond Oil - 36 g
- Neroli Essential Oil - .5 g

- Rose Absolute Essential Oil (Or a Substitute) - .5g
- Cosmetic Jar (Pet or Glass Jar) - 1
- Grapefruit Essential Oil - .5 g
- Vitamin E Oil - .75 g
- Isopropyl Myristate - 15 g

Where to Find Ingredients

These ingredients are readily available at any market near you, and although the ingredients were carefully chosen to give the body butter an air-like consistency, substitutes are available. If you can't find shea butter, you may substitute it with mango or avocado butter. They result in the same cloudy consistency, but they may feel grainy. You can also replace the sweet almond oil with any other lightweight oil like sunflower or grapeseed oil to give it the same light consistency. The Neroli and Rose essential oils can be substituted with sweet orange or other floral essential oil. The Isopropyl Myristate gives the non-greasy element to the body butter and can be substituted with any lightweight essential oil. However, it may not be able to give it the same light consistency.

Directions

1. First, weigh the refined shea butter and place it into the PET plastic, glass, or aluminum bowl.

2. Whisk the shea butter with an electric hand blender for 3-5 minutes until it is light and fluffy.

3. Blend the isopropyl myristate it into the mixture with the electric hand blender.

4. Then add the sweet almond essential oil and continue blending it until all ingredients are well blended.

5. Add the vitamin E oil to the mixture and blend.

6. Then put in the other essential oils and carefully blend for the last time until it has a cloud-like consistency and soft touch.

7. Make sure that your mixture is not too runny. If it is, check the measurements and try again.

8. Make sure that you don't whip your shea butter too much.

9. The mixture must not be too hard. If it is, you have added more shea butter than was required.

10. Put the mixture into containers.

Tips and Tricks
1.   Make sure you carefully check the measurements to keep the mixture from becoming too runny or too hard. 2.   The shelf life of this shea butter is around a year. You can extend it by adding more vitamin E oil.

Ingredient Substitutions	
Shea butter	Mango or avocado butter
Neroli/Rose essential oil	Sweet orange/ any floral essential oil
Essential oils - Sweet almond oil	Sunflower/Safflower oil/ any lightweight oil

Orange and Almond Whipped Body Butter

The store-bought body butter may not be the best choice for people with sensitive skin. There is a possibility that your skin may react to parabens or petroleum in store-bought products. This DIY whipped body butter consists of a mixture of orange and almond essential oils that adds a subtle aroma to the mixture, and it is pretty easy to make. The shea butter and coconut butter in the blend will make your skin feel nourished, soft, and hydrated.

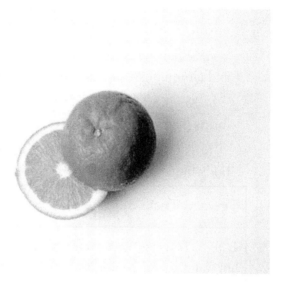

Ingredients

- Raw Shea Butter - 107 g
- Sweet Almond Oil - 54.7 g
- Orange Essential Oil - 0.99 g
- Almond Extract - 6.3 g
- Organic Coconut Oil - 54 g

Where to Find Ingredients

Most of these ingredients can be found in the nearest stores. However, raw cocoa butter can be substituted for shea butter. There are no substitutes for the almond and orange oils available as this recipe focuses explicitly on these two substances.

Directions

1. First, combine the shea butter, sweet almond oil, and coconut oil in a double boiler or a pot.

2. Keep stirring the ingredients in the bowl over medium-low heat until the ingredients melt.

3. Then remove the bowl from the heat and allow the mixture to cool down.

4. When the mixture has set, add in the essential oils and almond extract, and whip it until thoroughly mixed.

5. Keep whipping until the mixture turns soft and forms peaks.

6. Then add the mixture to containers and enjoy your body butter.

Tips and Tricks
1.   You can place your glass bowl in a bowl of hot water if you do not have a double boiler. 2.   Store it at room temperature.

Ingredient Substitutions	
Shea butter	Cocoa butter

Winter Skin Carrot Infused Body Butter

This winter skin carrot-infused body butter is wonderful for your skin to fight the winter season. This body butter is light and has a glossy look thanks to its lightweight essential oils and mango butter. It also has a great floral scent from the geranium and sandalwood essential oils. It also battles itchy and dry skin to help you get through the cold season. This homemade body butter is quite easy to make and will save you a lot of money, considering how cost-effective it is.

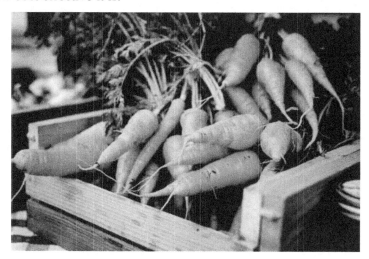

Ingredients

- Shea Butter - 48g
- Isopropyl Myristate - 15g
- Grapeseed Oil - 17g
- Vitamin E Oil - 1g
- Geranium Essential Oil - 5 drops
- Patchouli Essential Oil - 10 drops
- Carrot Infused Oil - 20g
- Sandalwood Essential Oil - 5 drops
- Mango Butter - 48g

Where to Find Ingredients

You can readily find these ingredients at any department store near you. If you have extremely dry skin, use shea butter in place of mango butter. You may substitute lightweight essential oils like grapeseed oil with other available lightweight essential oils. However, the essential oils used in this recipe give the end-product its color.

Directions

1. First, weigh the shea butter and the mango butter.

2. Then, whisk them until you are satisfied with the mixture's fluffiness and creaminess.

3. Add the Isopropyl myristate to the mixture and combine it.

4. Then, add the carrot and grapeseed oil into the mixture and whisk it.

5. The mango butter and shea butter may cause the mixture to become grainy. However, you can minimize the graininess by stirring it. Test it for grains by feeling it between your fingers.

6. Then add the vitamin E oil and essential oils into the mixture.

7. Whisk these ingredients until it becomes fluffy and soft.

8. Then you can place the body butter into the containers, and it is ready.

Tips and Tricks	
1. The recipe yields 150g body butter. However, you will need a 200g jar to make room for the fluffiness of the body butter.	
Ingredient Substitutions	
Mango butter	Shea butter
Grapeseed oil	Any other lightweight oil

Whipped Body Butter Recipe with Raspberry

This whipped raspberry body butter recipe is for you if you are not comfortable adding Isopropyl Myristate. It makes the body butter less greasy and uses arrowroot powder as its substitute. The arrowroot powder also makes the body butter thicker and brings in the magic of beneficial vitamins that make your skin feel smoother and softer. This recipe only uses heavy carrier oils, so it may feel a bit greasy despite the arrowroot powder. The body butter may be greasy, but it is best used after a shower as it may take some time to be absorbed into the skin. It is also excellent for massages.

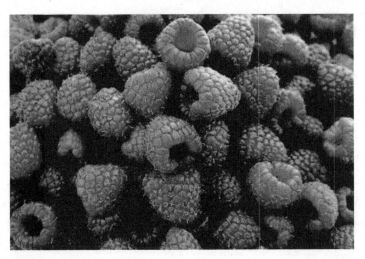

Ingredients

- Refined Shea Butter - 151g

- Arrowroot Powder - 6.5g

- Cornstarch - ½ cup or 64g

- Beetroot Powder - 0.7g

- Coconut Oil - 128g

- Raspberry Fragrance Oil - 1g

Where to Find Ingredients

These ingredients are readily available at your nearest market. If you want to use Isopropyl Myristate to substitute for arrowroot powder, then go for it. While arrowroot powder is a fantastic source for many wonderful vitamins, isopropyl myristate is better for making it less greasy. You can also use any other floral or fruity essential oil in place of raspberry essential oil. Moreover, you can also use mango or avocado butter instead of shea butter. However, it might make the body butter grainier.

Directions

1. First, weigh the shea butter and place it in a big bowl.

2. Then, whisk it on medium-low for 1-2 minutes until it becomes fluffy.

3. Melt the coconut oil in the microwave at shorter intervals to hinder it from heating up. Or you can also warm it in a water bath.

4. Then, blend the beetroot powder into the coconut oil and mix it with a frother or a small milk whisk. This helps disperse the powder into the mixture. It may form clumps in the mixture and cause it to become grainy. However, there is nothing to worry about as it will not affect the mixture's effectiveness.

5. Use a spatula to mix the coconut oil with shea butter. Then, move it back to the blender and blend the mixture at medium-low speed.

6. Add the arrowroot powder and the raspberry fragrance essential oil.

7. Gently mix the mixture and transfer it into the containers.

Tips and Tricks

1.　　This mixture will last up to 6 months. However, you can extend its shelf life by adding in vitamin E oil (at 1%) while adding the fragrance or some rosemary CO2 Extract at 0.1%.

Ingredient Substitutions

Arrowroot powder	Isopropyl Myristate
Raspberry fragrance oil	Other floral or fruity essential oil
Shea butter	Mango/avocado butter

Easy Body Butter Recipe with Jojoba Oil

This easy body butter is excellent as it helps make your skin feel smooth, nourished, and hydrated. It may seem greasy, but it is excellent for use after a shower. The natural softness of shea butter makes your skin feel soft and hydrated. The jojoba oil is an antibacterial, moisturizing, and oil-controlling carrier oil that is fabulous on the skin. You can use the anti-grease arrowroot flour starch to hinder the mixture from becoming greasy.

Ingredients

- Shea Butter unrefined/crude or refined - 41g

- Jojoba oil - 42g

- Lavender essential oil - 34 drops

- Arrowroot flour starch - 5g

- Mango butter (41g) or Cocoa butter (34g)

Where to Find Ingredients

These ingredients are readily available at any market near you. This recipe is easy to make, and substitutes are available for almost every ingredient. You can use mango butter or cocoa butter, whichever is available. You can also use any carrier oil in place of jojoba oil, such as almond oil. Moreover, use any essential oil as a substitute for the lavender essential oil and use Isopropyl Myristate in place of the arrowroot flour starch.

Directions

1. First, add shea butter and cocoa butter to a glass bowl.

2. Add some water to a saucepan and put it on heat. Then, place the glass bowl in the saucepan to melt the butter.

3. Add the arrowroot flour to the lavender essential oil in a separate bowl and whisk it.

4. Then remove the melted butter from the heat and add the jojoba oil and arrowroot flour mixture to the bowl with the melted butter and mix.

5. Allow the mixture to cool down for a few minutes, and then put it in the fridge to solidify it.

6. Remove the mixture from the fridge once it becomes opaque and feels firm.

7. Add the lavender essential oil to the mixture.

8. Use a whisk to blend the mixture until it looks smooth and whipped.

9. Once the body butter becomes fluffy, you may add it to the containers.

Tips and Tricks	
1. Store the mixture at room temperature and not directly under the sunlight. 2. You can increase its shelf life from 6 months and more by adding vitamin E oil.	
Ingredient Substitutions	
Cocoa butter	Mango butter (or vice versa)
Jojoba oil	Almond oil or any other carrier oil
Lavender essential oil	Any essential oil of your choice.

Whipped Gingerbread Body Butter

This whipped gingerbread body butter recipe is amazing for keeping your skin looking silky, smooth, and soft. It consists of a cinnamon-gingery scent that gives you major fall vibes. These scents also offer aromatherapy benefits that help calm your nerves and make you feel relaxed. The coconut oils, almonds, and shea butter make your skin hydrated, glowing, and silky-soft.

Ingredients

- Shea Butter Unrefined/Crude or Refined - 115g
- Almond Oil - 2 tbsp
- Coconut Oil- 54g
- Vitamin E - 2 tsp
- Ground Ginger - 2tsp
- Ground Cinnamon - 1 tsp
- Vanilla Extract 1 tsp

Where to Find Ingredients

These ingredients can be easily found at any market. This DIY body butter recipe is easy to make, and substitutes are available for almost every ingredient. You can use cocoa butter or mango butter in place of shea butter. You also have the option of using jojoba oil as a substitute for almond oil.

Directions

1. First, add shea butter, coconut oil, and almond oil to a microwave-safe glass bowl.

2. Place the bowl in the microwave and heat it in 30-second intervals. Stir between each interval until it melts and turns liquid.

3. Then take the mixture out of the microwave and let it cool down on the counter.

4. Once it is cool, place it in the refrigerator for 12 minutes until it becomes firm.

5. Then, add the cinnamon, vanilla extract, vitamin E, and ground ginger into the mixture and blend it well until it becomes fluffy and light.

6. Place the soft and fluffy mixture into jars or containers and close it tightly.

Tips and Tricks
1.   You can heat the butter mixture by placing the dish in a saucepan with hot water.   2.   You can keep the mixture in the refrigerator to keep it firm.

Ingredient Substitutions	
Shea butter	Mango butter or Cocoa butter
Jojoba oil	Almond oil or any other carrier oil

Double Chocolate Body Butter Recipe

This whipped double chocolate body butter recipe is a treat for chocolate lovers who also have an affiliation with natural products. This rich body butter is great for the winter season and will help moisturize your skin by giving it a smooth and silky glow.

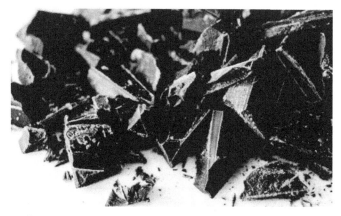

Ingredients

- Cocoa Butter - 120 g
- Almond Oil - 2 tbsp
- Pure Virgin Coconut Oil- 108g
- Beeswax Pastilles - 1 tsp
- Raw Cacao Powder - 1 ½ tbsp
- Pure Vanilla Extract - 1 tbsp

Where to Find Ingredients

These ingredients are quite commonly used and can be found at any department store.

Directions

1. First, add cocoa butter, coconut oil, and beeswax to a glass bowl and melt it in a microwave in 30-second intervals or place the bowl in boiling water in a saucepan.

2. Keep stirring the mixture until it melts.

3. Then, remove the mixture from the heat and add the almond oil, raw cacao powder, and pure vanilla extract.

4. Then carefully blend the mixture until it becomes fluffy.

5. Allow the mixture to cool down in a refrigerator for a few hours until it becomes firm.

6. Then blend the mixture again until it gets cloud-like consistency.

7. Once it becomes smooth, light, and fluffy, transfer the mixture to containers or jars.

Tips and Tricks	
1. You can also add peppermint essential oil to give it the chocolate-peppermint scent.	
Ingredient Substitutions	
Cocoa butter	Shea butter
Almond oil	Any other carrier oil

The body butter recipes discussed in this chapter are sensitive skin-friendly. Check the ingredients to ensure they don't contain any allergens or irritants that may trigger any reactions. These recipes are cost-effective, easy to make, and excellent to use. They consist of many beneficial properties that make your skin look smoother and more youthful. Experiment until you find the body butter recipe that best suits your skin and won't clog your pores.

Chapter 9: Preserving and Labeling Your Butters

We discussed in previous chapters the basic recipes and ingredients for homemade body butter for your body and face. Now we will discuss what comes after making the body butter, which is preserving, storing, and labeling your new product. Although homemade body butter is better than commercial ones because it doesn't contain any chemicals, it doesn't have a very long shelf life. Organic products don't usually last as long as commercial ones. Therefore, you have to store them properly to extend their shelf life.

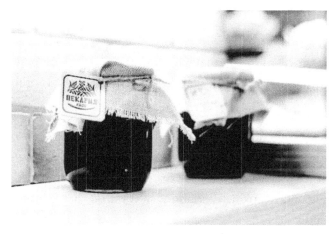

How to Preserve and Store Homemade Body Butter

Some of the ingredients you use may serve as a breeding ground for bacteria and other microorganisms. Without preservatives and proper storage, the body butter may go bad after a couple of weeks. Therefore, to avoid having any microbes growing in your product, you must add preservatives. Unpreserved products are dangerous, especially as you may not notice if they go bad. The body butter may become covered with yeast or mold, and you may not be able to tell because, for the most part, bacterial growth is invisible. If you don't preserve your product, you may end up with skin infections. Remember, you are making a natural and organic product to protect your skin at home. If left unpreserved, it will defeat its purpose and harm your skin.

It should be noted that homemade body butter doesn't last as long as commercial ones, even with preservatives. Luckily, there are natural preservatives available to protect your product and guarantee that you can enjoy it for a good few months. Preservatives will give it a longer shelf life, which isn't over 6 months. For this reason, we recommend that you don't make large quantities and make small batches that won't last over 6 months. However, if you happen to make large quantities, you can give them as gifts to family or friends, which they will surely enjoy.

Preserving and adequately storing your homemade body butter is vital for your health and others if you sell it or gift it.

Use Antioxidants

Adding antioxidants will slow down the oxidation process in some ingredients. Naturally, your product will be exposed to air every time you open the jar or container, compromising the ingredients and causing oxidation. Several oils act as antioxidants like rosemary and Vitamin E, so as a precaution, you shouldn't heat these oils directly.

Proper Storage

Proper storage will guarantee your body butter will have a long shelf life. Any homemade product, including body butter, should be stored in a dark place away from light. Also, keep it away from direct heat, so don't leave it in the sun. Additionally, make sure it is stored in a dry and cool place. Avoiding getting water in your body butter will also guarantee that it has a long shelf life. Therefore, don't use it when your hands are wet. If you want your body butter to remain soft, then make sure that you close it properly after every use.

Another thing recommended to ensure your product has a long shelf life and remains fresh is the container is to store the body butter in a glass jar. You don't have to buy an expensive or over-the-top glass jar, and you can simply opt for mason jars. Additionally, ensure the jar is watertight and airtight to keep air and moisture out. It also must have a lid that you shut tightly after every use. If you use preservatives and keep the product away from water, you won't have to worry about bacteria or mold, and your product will have an appropriate shelf life.

Use Clean Tools

Every tool you use to make the body butter must be clean to increase its shelf life. Therefore, you have to ensure that the jars, containers, tins, and bottles are all sterilized and clean. Whether you opt for new containers or use ones you already have at home, you have to wash them thoroughly with soap and water before using them. If you use a container or jar you already have, clean it thoroughly to ensure there aren't any particles or small bits of food in it.

Additionally, add a small amount of white vinegar while cleaning the container. White vinegar is a natural product that can kill certain bacteria. After cleaning the container, wait until it is completely dry before using it. You can use a dishwasher since it can clean and sterilize your tools. When storing your tools, make sure you keep them away from the kitchenware you use for making food. You should also wash your hands while making the body butter, and every time you use a tool, you won't introduce any new bacteria to your product.

The tips mentioned here will give the body butter an appropriate shelf life, and we recommend you use the product immediately and don't store it for too long, or the butter may lose its texture. It is better to use it while it is still fresh.

Protect It from Melting

After making your homemade body butter, you may notice it melts during the warm weather. You should fix this if you are planning to sell and ship your product. To ensure your body butter doesn't melt, you may have to reformulate the recipe, and increasing ingredients like cocoa butter, beeswax, or hard oils will do the trick. However, you should know that adding hard oils will prevent the body butter from quickly melting on your skin. On the other hand, it will make the body butter remain consistent at high temperature or use it after a hot shower.

Packaging

When choosing the packaging, the main thing that you should keep in mind is safety. It is essential to choose packaging that will protect your product. For this reason, it is best to choose a container. Additionally, you must ensure that your packaging doesn't affect your body butter composition. You can choose from various materials, but we recommend you use either stainless steel or glass. Stainless steel will work with any recipe, and glass won't allow any liquid or air to pass through and will not affect any ingredients. You can also opt for PET (polyethylene terephthalate) or HDPE (High-Density Polyethylene) containers since they are safe to use and, like glass, they also don't allow any liquid or air to pass through.

Additionally, PET and HDPE containers are made of plastic, so they won't break easily, and they will also protect your product from fluctuating temperatures.

In addition to the container's material, there are other things you should consider. You must make sure that the packaging allows you to use the product easily, especially if you want to sell it. Therefore, opt for packaging with a large diameter opening, so you can easily access and apply the body butter. Additionally, ensure the packaging is the right capacity or size and make sure that you aren't packaging too little or too much of the product.

Choosing the suitable packaging for your homemade body butter is essential for various reasons. First, as we have mentioned, choosing the right package will protect your product from different factors like air and temperature. The proper packaging will also guarantee that the body butter will have a long shelf life. Packaging will play a huge role in whether you plan on gifting or selling the body butter. If you plan to sell it, the packaging, if done correctly, will make a strong first impression and give it an advantage as it will attract customers. Additionally, it will make it easy for them to use and store it. If you plan to gift it, a nice packaging will show the recipient that you have put a lot of thought into your gift, making it more unique and personalized.

Alternatively, you can't choose just any packaging from the internet, especially if you are going to sell your product. Take your time and find packaging that reflects who you are and what your business is. Don't opt for something that has too many colors, as it can be distracting and put the customer off. Additionally, don't go for something too complicated to use. This is a body butter container, and people want to open it easily, use it, and close it as simply as possible. You have probably used commercial body butter before, so ask yourself, what attracted you to the packaging? What type of packaging has put you off? Think of what you like about the body butter packaging you bought, so you can apply it to yours and avoid what you don't like. However, it is vital that you don't copy another product's packaging because this can get you in legal trouble.

Some people prefer to use expensive packaging because they want to use something pretty for their product. You don't have to opt for expensive. You can find various attractive packaging at reasonable prices. The lid is also an important part of the packaging for two reasons: first, it protects the product from air and moisture when it is shut tightly. Secondly, lids come in different colors and shapes that will appeal to the recipients of your gifts or will attract customers if you choose to sell your products. Last but not least, every business has a message it wants to convey through packaging, like eco-friendly businesses that don't use plastic. Make sure you determine your new business's message initially so that you can use packaging that reflects it.

Labeling

Labeling your homemade body butter is a very important step. If the packaging is used to make a first impression, then the labeling is how you introduce your product. You should include what your product is using in clear and simple words to avoid confusion in your label. This is body butter, a product, so you must write this on the label. You can't write lotion and expect that people won't know the difference. Lotions and body butter are two very different products, so be clear and specific. The labeling should also be written in large font and placed on the front of the body butter package.

Additionally, it must include all the ingredients; this is crucial you sell or gift your product. You need to mention all the ingredients you used in the body butter. Accuracy is key. Usually, people check the list of ingredients on any product to ensure that it is safe and there isn't any ingredient they are allergic to. If you forget or choose not to include one ingredient and someone uses the product and gets an allergy reaction, they will have grounds to sue you and possibly ruin your reputation. Therefore, you must include all the ingredients. It is better to be safe than sorry. Also, list the ingredients from the most to least used.

In addition to the ingredients, include the manufacture date, the shelf life, and the product's expiration date. It will give your body butter credibility. It is also recommended to include the quantity of the body butter in millimeters or ounces on the label. This information will make the product appear legit, so people will trust it and be inclined to use it. No one will use a product with no information written on it. Since many body products are made with ingredients like coconut, shea butter, and strawberry, you should include a warning label that this product isn't edible. You may think that people will know better than to consume these products, but this warning will absolve you from any responsibility if someone does consume them. Also, include that the product is for external use only and whether the body butter is for the face or the body.

Additionally, since many people now prefer to use vegan or cruelty-free products not tested on animals, consider adding this piece of information, too, but only if it is true. If you haven't used any animal-based products, you can include that the product is vegan. Only include the words cruelty-free if neither the products nor any ingredients were tested on animals. Properly labeling your body butter will protect you and the people using your product. Therefore, take your time and use correct and accurate information.

The design of the label is also important. Just like packaging, you can't copy another product's label, or you will get in trouble. In this case, Pinterest is your best friend. Whether you plan on designing it yourself or hire someone to do the job for you, you will most likely find a multitude of designs on the app, and you can use them as inspiration.

Making homemade body butter is a fun DIY project allowing you to make a safe and organic product that won't harm your skin. Many people have made a business selling their organic products. If you want to do the same, there are certain cosmetic laws and guidelines you should be aware of and abide by to avoid any legal trouble.

International Cosmetic Laws Briefing

To be safe and sell your product to the public, you should follow the FDA regulations. Before we go any further, we must advise you to research the international cosmetic laws and regulations before selling or gifting your product to avoid any legal issues.

Since you are making an organic product, you will most likely want to add the word "organic" to its label. However, know that the FDA regulates using this word. Your body butter must include a certain percentage of organic ingredients to be qualified as organic by the FDA. So, first, check the FDA website to learn about the percentages before using the term organic on your label. The FDA is very strict about labeling, and you must adhere to its standards. For instance, if you want to mention on your label that your product "isn't tested on animals," then you should first check the FDA definition of animal testing. The FDA also has serious requirements regarding a product's shelf life and expiration. Therefore, it is vital that your product is tested for stability according to the FDA regulations before including this piece of information. Additionally, all the ingredients you use must be considered safe for use under the FD&C Act.

So, any information you include on your label must follow FDA laws and regulations. To avoid any legal trouble, check the FDA website for their standards on every piece of information you plan to include in your label.

Chapter 10: How to Use Your Body Butter

As mentioned in a previous chapter, body butter, although majorly used to moisturize your skin, is used for many other moisturizing needs. Now that you've learned how to make body butter at home, it is essential to learn how to use it properly. In addition to using a suitable recipe, whether for your hair or nails, you also need to ensure you're using the product correctly, or it won't have the expected desirable results. This chapter will walk you through the various ways to use body butter, with step-by-step instructions to ensure you don't make mistakes.

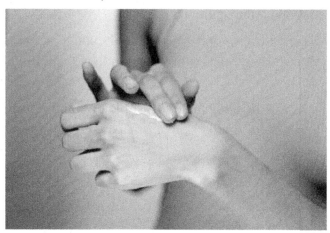

All-Body Moisturizing

Body butter is usually thicker than the usual lotions and creams and is more moisturizing for your skin. If you want to lock the moisture into your skin, the best time to use body butter would be right after your daily shower or bath. If you have dry skin, use body butter daily after every shower. But, if your skin is oily, use body butter only 2-3 times a week.

Step-by-Step Guide

Follow these instructions to ensure proper use of the product without wasting.

1. After your daily bath, use a clean towel to pat your body dry, but don't dry your body completely. Instead, leave some moisture remaining.

2. Take a dime-sized amount of body butter and apply it to your skin in firm board strokes. You can use your fingers or a spatula to apply.

3. Wait a few seconds to let the butter melt on your skin. The natural heat from your body will melt the butter on your skin, making it easier to absorb.

4. With the palms of your hands, rub the butter onto your skin in long, firm strokes until the body butter is smoothed into a thin layer.

5. Add a second layer of body butter to spots dryer than others, like your knees, elbows, and other dry patches.

6. Let the body butter dry for a few minutes before you get dressed. If your skin appears too greasy, wipe it with a towel.

Do's and Don'ts

- Don't leave your skin too wet. Otherwise, it will be hard to smooth it onto your skin as the butter will interact with water.

- Use a spatula to apply the body butter onto your skin so that you don't contaminate the container with your hands.

- Don't apply too much product as it contains butter and oil and will make your skin look greasy.

- Wait a few seconds after applying body butter before putting clothes on as it might leave oily stains on your clothes.

Warnings

- Make sure you check the ingredients in the body butter product you're using. Avoid retinol, alpha-hydroxy acid, and artificial fragrances.

- Natural body butter has essential oil blends, so be sure to check if you're allergic to any ingredients.

For Hair Revitalization

You can use body butter to moisturize and nourish dry and damaged hair. Similar to how body butter helps hydrate your skin, it can also hydrate dry hair that lacks moisture. Dry hair can quickly turn frizzy, coarse, and brittle if left untreated. Body butter, specially formulated for your hair, contains natural oils and many other hydrating ingredients that nourish dry and damaged hair.

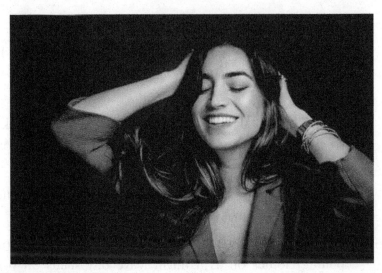

Step-by-Step Guide

Follow these instructions to ensure proper use of the product without wasting.

As a Hair Mask

1. Apply shampoo to your hair and rinse well.

2. Apply a leave-in conditioner or any other product you use.

3. Take a dollop of body butter and apply it to your damp scalp and strands. Massage it into your hair with the tips of your fingers.

4. If you have dry hair, leave it on for an hour, and then wash it out.

5. For curly hair, leave the body butter hair mask on overnight and wash it off in the morning.

As a Leave-In Conditioner

1. After shampooing your hair, take a pea-sized amount of body butter.

2. Apply from mid-length to the ends of your hair, either dry or damp.

3. Don't wash your hair after the application.

As a Pre-Conditioner

1.   Apply the body butter to the damp ends of your hair, massage the product into the hair ends and not the scalp.

2.   Leave the butter on for about an hour, then rinse it off with a mild shampoo.

Do's and Don'ts

Do's

• Wash your hair with lukewarm water before applying body butter to your hair, as this opens the cuticles and allows better absorption.

• Use body butter on damp or wet hair to maximize its effect.

• When applying body butter to your hair, focus on the ends of your hair rather than the scalp.

• Apply body butter only to clean hair. Otherwise, the dirt and butter will react, build up, and lead to hair fall.

Don'ts

• Never reapply butter unless you've washed off the residue from the previous application.

• Body butter contains ingredients that can weigh your hair down. So, if you have thin hair, don't use body butter excessively.

• Don't combine body butter with hair products like gels and mousses because they will make your hair look exceptionally greasy.

Warnings

Ensure that you use specially designed body butter meant for your hair. Otherwise, the product's harmful oils and ingredients (for your hair) may damage your hair.

As Makeup Remover

Body butter can also be used as a natural makeup remover because it contains oleic acid as an ingredient. The shea butter deep conditions the skin and leaves it soft and smooth.

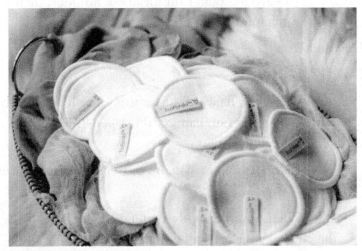

Step-by-Step Guide

Follow these instructions to ensure proper use of the product without wasting.

1. Take a dime-sized amount of body butter out of its container and let it melt on the palm of your hands.

2. Once melted, use a cotton ball or pad to apply the butter to your skin. Spread it evenly and absorb it into your skin.

3. Gently but firmly, wipe the makeup from your skin with the cotton pad containing the body butter product.

4. Rub until the last traces of makeup products are removed from your skin, then wash your face.

5. Reapply a coat of body butter after rinsing your face for extra conditioning.

Do's and Don'ts

• Do not rub off your makeup too harshly, as it can damage your skin.

• Use a cotton pad to absorb and apply the body butter to your face for best results. If not available, you can use wipes or plain cotton.

• Don't apply excessive product to your face as it could clog your pores and form pimples. It is important to rinse your face after using body butter to remove makeup.

Warnings

• Natural body butter has essential oil blends, so be sure to check if you're allergic to any ingredients.

To Treat Eczema

Body butter formulated to treat eczema and other skin irritations contain ingredients that provide anti-inflammatory properties. These properties help treat eczema, pain, and irritation. Body butter gets absorbed quickly and moisturizes the epidermis layer when applied to your skin.

Step-by-step guide

Follow these instructions to ensure proper use of the product without wasting.

1. Take a warm bath or shower, and pat your skin dry, leaving some moisture remaining.

2. Apply the usual dime-sized amount of body butter to your whole body with your palms or a spatula.

3. Rub the body butter into your skin in long, broad strokes until completely absorbed. Let it dry for a while.

4. Now, reapply a new coat of eczema treating body butter onto the spots affected by eczema. You can use

more than the usual amount of body butter here to ensure maximum nourishment.

5. Let the body butter dry for a few minutes before you get dressed. If your skin appears too greasy, wipe it with a towel.

Do's and Don'ts

• Don't leave your skin too wet. Otherwise, it will be hard to smooth as the butter will interact with the water.

• Use a spatula to apply the body butter onto your skin so that you don't contaminate the container with your hands.

• Shower twice a day and follow the same application procedure for the best results.

• Don't scratch the sensitive eczema areas when applying the butter.

• Make sure not to touch other parts of your body not exposed to eczema after application.

• Don't apply too much product as it contains butter and oil and will make your skin look greasy.

Warnings

• Make sure you check the ingredients in the body butter product you're using. Avoid retinol, alpha-hydroxy acid, and artificial fragrances.

• Consult your doctor before using any products to treat a skin disease, like eczema, as allergic reactions may occur.

Treating Dry Hands and Feet Overnight

Some spots on your body are usually dryer than others, and these include your knees, elbows, hands, feet, and similar areas. A great way to use body butter is to apply it to your dry areas for an overnight moisturizing treatment. For this type of treatment, it is advisable to use thicker body butter than usual for increased nourishment. This butter is extremely moisturizing and can help heal even cracked skin.

Step-by-Step Guide

Follow these instructions to ensure proper use of the product without wasting.

1. Before your bedtime, apply a thin layer of butter to your feet.

2. Start with a dime-sized amount, and add more as needed.

3. Add extra butter to dry areas, especially your ankle joints.

4. Using long, firm strokes, massage the butter entirely onto your feet.

5. The butter should melt on your skin and absorb into it automatically.

6. Wait a few seconds for your feet to dry, then put on socks, and you can also put your socks on while the product is still drying. Although this will stain your socks, it does provide an intense treatment because the socks lock the moisture in.

7. Next, repeat the same process on your hands and put on gloves to lock the moisture into your hands.

8. Remove your socks and gloves in the morning, and you'll find your skin feeling soft, moisturized, and healed.

Do's and Don'ts

• Don't leave your skin too wet. Otherwise, it will be hard to smooth as the butter will interact with water.

• Don't apply too much product as it contains butter and oil and will make your skin look greasy.

- Natural body butter has essential oil blends, so be sure to check if you're allergic to any ingredients.

To Treat Cellulite

Body butter is excellent for healing your skin. Body butter formulated to heal stretch marks, cellulite, and scars are usually thicker than the usual lotions and creams and are more moisturizing to your skin. They also contain vitamin E and a blend of moisturizing butter. If you want to lock the moisture into your skin, the best time to use body butter would be right after your daily shower or bath.

Step-by-Step Guide

Follow these instructions to ensure proper use of the product without wasting.

1. After your daily bath, use a clean towel to pat your body dry but don't dry your body completely. Instead, leave some moisture remaining.

2. Scoop out a pea-sized amount of body butter with your fingers. Although you can use more than this amount, it is advisable to start small and keep adding more if needed.

3. Rub the lotion between the palms of your hands to melt it. It will only take a few seconds for the body butter to melt from your body heat.

4. Apply the butter to the affected area and gently rub it using firm, circular motions. Add more if needed.

5. Wait a few minutes for the butter to dry before covering your skin.

Do's and Don'ts

• Don't use body butter excessively, as it will make your skin look greasy.

- Wipe off any excess butter from the affected area before covering it with clothes.

- You can apply extra body butter to chapped or damaged skin to heal it faster.

Warnings

- Test the body butter on a patch of skin first before applying it to sensitive areas of your body to avoid allergic reactions.

- Make sure you check the ingredients in the body butter product you're using. Avoid retinol, alpha-hydroxy acid, and artificial fragrances.

- Natural body butter has essential oil blends, so be sure to check if you're allergic to any ingredients.

For Locking in Fragrance

One of the best uses of body butter is its ability to help your perfume last all day long. The combination of butter and oils in these products makes them a perfect base for your fragrance to adhere to. Plus, they lock the fragrance of your perfume in and enhance the scent through the essential oil blends they contain. So, if you want to smell lovely all day without having to reapply perfume every second, use the body butter product that goes well with your perfume.

Step-by-step guide

Follow these instructions to ensure proper use of the product without wasting.

1. After your morning shower, pat yourself with a towel but don't dry your skin completely.

2. When your skin is dewy, take a small amount of body butter into your hands and let it melt in your palm.

3. Apply the melted butter onto your skin, and rub it to help it get absorbed completely.

4. At this point, apply your fragrance or perfume to your body when the body butter still hasn't dried (it has a greasy, wet look).

5. Wait a few seconds for the perfume to attach to the butter particles, and let both dry.

Do's and Don'ts

• Don't wait for the butter to dry, and then apply your perfume. Otherwise, the fragrance effect will be nullified.

• Don't leave your skin too wet because it will be hard to smooth it as the butter will interact with water.

• Combine your perfume with a body butter having the same or similar scent that compliments your perfume's fragrance.

• Don't use scented body butter if you have a skin condition, as it will only worsen the condition.

• Don't apply too much product as it contains butter and oil and will make your skin look greasy.

• Wait a few seconds before putting clothes on after applying body butter as it might leave oily stains on your clothes.

Warnings

• Scented body butter contains essential oils. While many of them are unreactive, the reactivity varies from person to person. So, if you're allergic or may be allergic to one of the essential oils, do a patch test prior to use.

• Make sure you check the ingredients in the body butter product you're using. Avoid retinol, alpha-hydroxy acid, and artificial fragrances that cause skin irritation.

Conclusion

This book aims to provide everything you need to create homemade and natural body butter. We started by mentioning the basics of body butter and that it is better to make them at home instead of buying them from a store. In the first chapter, we provided a brief history and listed the benefits of body butter. The second chapter explained the main ingredients of body butter to use as a base for your product. We provided details about the benefits of each ingredient and differentiated between the refined and unrefined forms of each one.

In the third chapter, we discussed the two main whipping techniques used to make body butter. We provided step-by-step procedures on how to create body butter using each technique. We also added a few tips to avoid malfunctions and gave example recipes for each technique. The fourth chapter highlighted the importance of choosing suitable essential oils for each recipe. It is essential to note the safety precautions before using certain essential oils for pregnant women or children. We discussed the properties and benefits of each oil and how to use them in your body butter recipes.

The fifth chapter was dedicated to basic recipes that we encourage you to start with. We provided a detailed description of each recipe, and a summary of each body butter's properties, a list of ingredients and where to find them, clear steps on how to execute the recipe, and different tips and tricks for substitutions and what to do if something goes wrong in the recipe.

The sixth chapter listed more difficult body butter recipes that included more ingredients but are undoubtedly worth trying once you get the hang of the basic recipes. The seventh chapter listed body butter recipes for specific conditions, like eczema, sun damage, aging, and cellulite, among others.

The eighth chapter was aimed at body butter recipes for the face, for use as either face masks or moisturizers. It is important to note that not all body butter can be used on your face. They should be made specifically for the face because it is more sensitive than the rest of the body.

The ninth chapter discussed an important step at the end of your process: knowing how to package, store, and label your product. It is imperative because organic products need to be handled with care to avoid spoilage due to a lack of preservatives. The final chapter mentioned the safest ways to use your homemade body butter for maximum effects. We also included a do's and don'ts section to consider before using your product on your skin to avoid any bad skin reactions. It is crucial to verify whether you can use the products on your skin with your doctor. We hope the book served as the perfect guide for creating your homemade and natural body butter.

Part 3: Bath Bombs

The Ultimate DIY Guide on How to Make Your Own Natural and Homemade Bath Bomb

Includes Simple and Organic Recipes

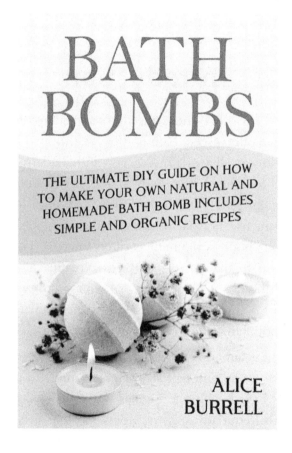

BATH BOMBS

THE ULTIMATE DIY GUIDE ON HOW TO MAKE YOUR OWN NATURAL AND HOMEMADE BATH BOMB INCLUDES SIMPLE AND ORGANIC RECIPES

ALICE BURRELL

Introduction

Have you ever watched those mesmerizing videos showing what happens when effervescent bath bombs are dropped in water and wondered how it all works? Are you intrigued by the vibrant colors and looking forward to trying them out? Are you interested in making your bath bombs at home, and did you know you can use normal household ingredients? If that's the case, then this book is definitely written for you! This book will introduce you to the sensory world of creating all-natural and organic bath bombs in the comfort of your own home. You will learn how to enjoy luxurious spa treatments in your own cozy bathtub without having to step foot out of the house!

This book is aimed at beginners interested in sustainable self-care products – and among them – bath bombs. In recent years, bath bombs have become a popular way to administer self-care, and they are frequently seen in videos posted on social media platforms. It is no surprise because everybody enjoys the wonderful colors that explode as soon as the bath bombs hit the water. This magical transformation is not just pleasing to the eyes. You will discover how bath bombs can tickle most of your senses and create a soothing and relaxing atmosphere.

We will discover how bath bombs are used for various purposes and what different ingredients are incorporated to induce a certain mood depending on the time of day. You will discover step-by-step procedures starting from drawing the perfect bath to creating a relaxing and romantic atmosphere and how to create your own bath bombs. You will be able to experiment with different essential oils and fragrances according to your personal preferences.

Nowadays, more people are looking for do-it-yourself recipes to make their own cosmetics, beauty products, and self-care items. Bath bombs are no different because they serve as the ultimate self-care product. In the following chapters, you will learn the basics of creating bath bombs and how you can play around with the ingredients to make a unique product. You will learn what tools and equipment you will need to conduct your experiments and what items are safe for use so that you can enjoy your baths every day.

You will also learn to make bath bombs for your kids using kid-friendly ingredients. We'll also teach you about different skin types and how to choose the most suitable ingredients for your skin. And in no time at all, you will be crafting a safe, sustainable, and cost-effective product at home.

Finally, we will suggest storing your creations for later use or packaging them as gifts. So, you'll be able to make large batches and not run out. Whether you love to make your own products or want to give them a try for the first time, this book will suit your needs. So, let's dive into the world of bath bombs and teach you how to make your own at home.

Chapter 1: Introduction to Bath Bombs

People usually have one of two types of baths. The most common one is taking a quick daily shower. The second type is the more luxurious form of bath that involves filling a tub with hot water and mixing in a few essential oils and effervescent granules that promote relaxation. Bath bomb art has been trending recently on social media, with people showing a renewed interest in bath time delights. However, the origin of bath bombs goes back for more than 30 years. This chapter will introduce you to the history of bath bombs. You will also learn about the benefits of using them and how to use them in your bath.

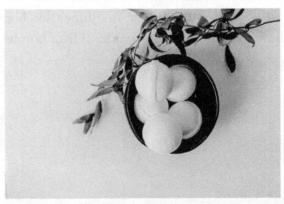

The Invention of Bath Bombs

Bath bombs are composed of essential oils, scents, and coloring pigments mixed and then molded into various shapes, but the most common shape is a ball which is why they have been dubbed "bath bombs." The purpose of a bath bomb is to create a luxurious experience far beyond simply drawing a bath and adding a mixture of essential oils. Dropping a bath bomb into a tub of hot water creates an effervescent reaction filled with color and fragrance, which is extremely eye-pleasing and makes you want to jump right in.

In 1989, the co-founder of Lush, a cosmetics company specializing in hand-made products, and product-inventor, Mo Constantine, came up with the idea of bath bombs to change the standard bath into a luxurious experience. Not only was the mundane bath experience to change, but Mo also wanted to create a product suitable for all types of skin and that causes zero irritation and at the same time elevates a daily routine into something special.

In the beginning, she experimented with cocoa butter bath bombs and continued developing the product until she was able to incorporate different colors and ingredients. Talking about the process, she said: *"I wanted to be able to introduce things to the bath which you wouldn't normally be able to, such as peels, petals, butter, and essential oils, lovely ingredients which would be beneficial to the skin."* The idea for the "fizzing" was inspired by watching the reaction of effervescent antacid tablets when they were put into water. The product which evolved after that was something that Mo Constantine never imagined. She wanted to create a product with ingredients found in any household.

People started posting videos of bath bombs in action – the effects of the bombs as they are dropped into a bathtub filled with hot water. The mesmerizing effect of them dissolving in water became a trend on all platforms. The product was further developed by Mo's son, Jack Constantine, who created a more complicated form of a bomb that had intricate, colorful patterns. His concept was to create a bath bomb with added benefits for the skin and something that customers could look forward to at the end of a long day. Bath bombs have now evolved to include enriching oils and body butter along with refreshing and luxurious scents and colors.

The aim was for people to feel that they were engaging in a work of art and not just a normal bath. Each bath bomb is unique, as you hardly ever get the same reaction from any given bath bomb, even if they have similar colors. The process of creating bath bombs involves a ton of experiments with all sorts of ingredients that may even include popping candy. The whole experience was aimed at making you feel relaxed and happy. Bath bombs were then grown and evolved into jelly bombs, which are used similarly but introduce a jelly-like substance in your bath. The special jelly coats your skin and leaves it feeling smoother than ever.

Bath bombs can include various ingredients such as Epsom salts that are used to relieve pain in sore muscles, which is why they are often recommended to be used after a workout session to help soothe your muscles. With the addition of essential oils and sweet almond oil, your skin is nourished and will stay fresh and hydrated. Lavender and lemongrass oils are also added for their soft, gentle fragrances and soothing effects. These are the core ingredients for the therapeutic version of bath bombs.

The effervescence reaction produced as the bath bomb hits the water results from baking soda and citric acid included in the ingredients, as well as sodium lauryl sulfoacetate that makes the bathwater foamier and more vibrant. Sodium lauryl sulfoacetate is used because of its organic origin in coconut oil. When Lush first introduced bath bombs, the company marketed them as containing only natural colorings and vegetarian products. Some bath bombs dissolve a lot slower than others because of the added layer of bubble bar mixture produced by Lush. They also use sustainable glitter that doesn't leave a residue as other craft glitters do. This means these bombs are completely environmentally-friendly, and you won't have to worry about glitter particles stuck all over your bathtub after you have finished.

Bath bombs are made by a hand-pressing technique, in which baking soda is mixed with colorings and fragrances depending on the type of bath bomb being made. This process is carefully carried out by a team of factory workers, who produce hundreds of bath bombs every single day. Every type of skin is accommodated for. Sensitive skin bombs contain various soothing essential oils like lavender and chamomile. Some versions do not contain any colorings or fragrances for people with extra sensitive skin. The sole purpose of adding coloring dyes is to play a major role in elevating your mood as you watch the frizzy reactions bursting with color in your bathtub.

How to Use Bath Bombs

While using a bath bomb might seem quite basic, there are a few tricks to make the experience reach its fullest potential. First, start by filling your tub all the way before you drop your bath bomb. If you're going to use extra items such as a bubble bar to create a foamier solution with plenty of bubbles, make sure you put it under running water. That way, you will ensure you get the most out of your bubble bar, rather than just dropping it in the water.

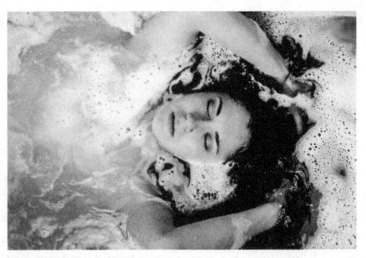

Make sure the water is as warm as your skin can tolerate. A hot bath helps you feel more relaxed and soothes your sore muscles, and it will help dissolve all the body butters in your chosen bath bomb to make sure that you are getting the best out of all the ingredients as intended. There is no set heating point for a bath because it is different for everyone, depending on your skin's sensitivity and how hot you prefer your bath. The temperature of your bath water also depends on how long you want to stay in your bath before the water starts to get cold. If you start the water a little hotter than you like, it will last you a lot longer. You could still add hot water if your bath cools too quickly. Make sure you don't draw a bath that is too hot because it may make you feel weak and exhausted. The idea is to give yourself a fragrant, wonderful experience in a relaxing bath, so it is important not to overdo it.

You can have as many additions as you want in your bath. While a typical bath bomb may be enough to relax you, you can also add an extra bubble bar and other bath oils to make the bath even more luxurious and vibrant. Every bath you create is your own sensual sanctuary and work of art. It is an excellent place to experiment with different products to make your combination.

Depending on the desired effect, add products that promote that feeling you are looking forward to the feeling when taking a bath. You can add calming essential oils such as lavender and chamomile if you want a regular relaxing bath. For a refreshing bath, use rose, lavender, or lemon oil in your bath or even a combination of all three. This combination should help make you feel refreshed for the whole day, and it is a perfect way to start your weekend when you have enough time for a long soak and still have time for the special activities you're looking forward to. Some bath mixtures to help relieve stress use ingredients that include bergamot, orange, and clary oils. These help to soothe your nerves and make you feel calmer, which is perfect after a long day at work. There are also special mixtures for more romantic nights, including fragrances like rose oils and vanilla powder.

Before even drawing a bath, decide on what kind of bath you feel like. Ask yourself if you would prefer a regular relaxing bath, a bath that will help you fall asleep, or a bath that will invigorate your senses and leave you feeling refreshed all day. Your bath can be as short or as long as you want to depend on your schedule. You can create a bath that is aimed to give you a revitalizing treatment like you would get in a spa. For this purpose, you can use lemongrass and ginger oils. No matter what outcome you want, you will find a bath bomb that is specific to that purpose. Invest in a few bath bombs and essential oils for every mood and create your own customized baths.

If you have extra sensitive skin, choose ingredients that won't irritate your skin, especially in combination with hot water, which might cause a skin rash. Use lukewarm water that is gentler on sensitive skin and soothing ingredients like oat milk and chamomile in your bath. Always check the ingredients on the bath bomb package to make sure it is suitable for your type of skin.

There is more to creating the perfect bath than just dropping a bath bomb. Creating the right setting for yourself will put you in a better mood and achieve the desired results. Ensure that your bathroom is decluttered so that your eyes *don't* fall on something that may bother you or make you think of the things you need to do. A bath is a place where you let your worries go, so it is best to create a relaxing atmosphere before you jump in. Get your bathrobe ready and choose your fluffiest towels and bath slippers to dry yourself after your bath. It is not a good idea to use a rough towel on your soft skin after the bath. Use the perfect light setting or light a few candles to create a relaxing mood. You can also put on some of your favorite music that helps you to relax. Think of your bath as a spa treatment by thinking about all of the steps ahead of your bath.

Why DIY Bath Bombs Are Better than Store-Bought Ones

The best types of bath bombs are the organic ones you can make at home. No matter how organic or natural ingredients are marketed for different bath bomb products, there will always be other synthetic materials and chemicals added. Synthetic fragrances are usually used in bath bombs to give a pleasing scent to attract customers. When you make your own bath bombs at home, you can guarantee that no chemical toxins are added.

While some companies use organic ingredients and less harmful substances, others use chemicals like sodium lauryl sulfate that causes skin irritation and other health problems. Many labels on bath bombs will mention fragrances in their ingredients list without mentioning the type of fragrance used. These fragrances are usually chemicals that are harmful to the body with repetitive use. A common fragrance like lilac is frequently used in bath bombs, and this has many harmful effects as it causes irritation and rashes to the skin. Other chemicals like phthalates are also used as a fragrance and cause hormonal imbalances, allergies, and other major side effects.

Many bath bombs in the market have artificial ingredients that do the opposite of moisturizing your skin. The synthetic materials in bath bombs remove the natural oils in your skin instead of retaining moisture, which results in dry skin that leads to irritation, rashes, and potential infections.

Some of the common ingredients present in commercial bath bombs, in addition to artificial fragrances, are coloring dyes, talc powder, and other additives. As mentioned, fragrances can include a wide range of scents for adults and kids like flowers, mint, cotton candy, and gum. Companies don't often state the type of fragrance, so you may be using harmful chemicals without even knowing. They could use natural dyes in combination with synthetic dyes, which, with repeated use, can affect your skin. You may be susceptible to skin irritations from synthetic dyes used in these products.

Bear in mind that even some natural ingredients may irritate more sensitive areas in your body, like your genitals. Talc powder is especially harmful to your reproductive system as it may travel to the ovaries and may lead to ovarian cancer. Some companies use plastic-based glitter particles and microbeads, which are not eco-friendly, so it is best not to use bath bombs that contain glitter or only use the non-plastic type.

The safest way to test a bath bomb is to rub it against your elbow and wait two days to see if your skin develops a bad reaction. A good rule of thumb is to keep your bath to 15 to 20 minutes maximum to avoid any allergic reaction. It is also important to rinse the excess products from your skin after taking a bath to remove any residue that could cause skin irritation. Ideally, limit using store-bought bath bombs to two or three times per week to avoid any harmful side effects.

It is best to create your own bath bomb at home to avoid the aforementioned potential adverse effects. When you create your own bath bomb, only use organic ingredients that will help keep your skin hydrated throughout the day. Recommended ingredients include olive oil, coconut oil, and citrus oils like lemon, orange, bergamot, and grapefruit.

The Benefits of Bath Bombs

When properly made, bath bombs are vegan-friendly and all-natural, making them sustainable, eco-friendly products that benefit both you and the environment. The natural and organic ingredients included won't give you skin irritations, redness, or potential infections. They should leave your skin rejuvenated because of their soothing and hydrating properties. And you'll have the added satisfaction of knowing that you created something beautiful and nourishing.

Home-crafted bath bombs usually include ingredients that moisturize all skin types. Softeners and emollients like cocoa butter and shea butter are common ingredients and work wonders for your skin, leaving it smooth and shiny. This is what makes bath bombs the perfect product for a luxurious bath. They also contain ingredients that cleanse your skin and help pamper your whole body as if you are getting a spa treatment. You don't have to worry about moisturizing each part of your body by itself. With one bath, you will be able to cleanse your body thoroughly and moisturize it at the same time.

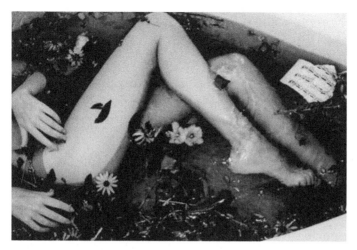

While bath bombs have a variety of ingredients, they usually contain two main items. The base of bath bombs consists of citric acid and baking soda or sodium bicarbonate, both of which are responsible for the effervescent reaction when exposed to water. They provide multiple good health effects, as they promote healing and repairing of the skin by helping to increase blood circulation. They also work to cleanse the body from all impurities and toxins and at the same time remove any bad odors from the body produced by bacteria from sweating. Their bubbling and fizzing action helps to provide healthy-looking skin and keeps it looking younger and refreshed.

A bath bomb is essentially a way to make your bath luxurious. Just looking at the vibrant colors and the soothing sound of the effervescent reaction, and you will instantly feel happier and more relaxed. The wonderful fragrances added will surround your senses, making you feel luxuriously pampered. A bath bomb is perfect and one of the easiest recipes for self-care, as all you need to do is drop your bath bomb in hot water and watch it bubble up.

The fragrances added to the bath bombs also double up and work as an aromatherapy session. The wonderfully soft and sensuous scents will remain with you throughout the day. By choosing a specific bath bomb for each time of the day, you will be able to enjoy the desired effect from your bath. A bath bomb helps to tickle your senses – from seeing the colorful foamy water, smelling the aromatic essential oils, and hearing the frizzy effervescent reaction to feeling the smooth bathwater on your skin, which creates the most well-rounded, relaxing, and joyful experience.

You don't need to wait to purchase a bath bomb from the store or online. You can get started right now in creating your own at home using ingredients that can easily be found in your kitchen or dressing table. You can get as creative as you want while mixing and matching different essential oils and natural fragrances to create a bath bomb for every mood. In a few simple steps, you will learn how to customize your own bath bombs according to how you feel or what takes your fancy. Creating personal bath bombs is far better for you if you intend to use them on a daily basis because you will guarantee that no toxic chemicals are added.

In this chapter, we introduced you to the world of bath bombs by mentioning their history and origins. We also gave you a few tips to create the perfect bath and bath bomb experience, together with the main benefits of using bath bombs. As we discussed above, there are so many advantages to creating your own bath bombs. It is the safest way to ensure the best bath experience possible, which you can enjoy every day. We encourage you to use this information to get started in creating your own bath bomb recipes, as will be further discussed in the upcoming chapters.

Chapter 2: Tools and Basic Ingredients

In the last chapter, we discussed the role of bath bombs and explained why it's better to make them at home than to buy commercial ones. In this chapter, we will discuss what goes into the making of homemade organic bath bombs and the tools and basic ingredients that you will need. Making bath bombs at home is a lot like cooking. It requires certain tools, ingredients, and recipes. It is an easy and fun DIY project that you will enjoy doing alone or with the help of your friends or kids. Once you get the right tools and prepare the ingredients, it won't take you longer than ten minutes to make your organic bath bombs.

The Tools

Mixing Bowl

The first thing that you will need is a mixing bowl to mix all the ingredients in. Preferably keep this separate from your cooking equipment.

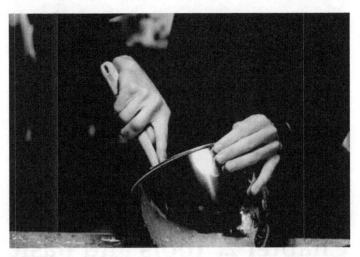

Whisk

Another vital tool you'll need is a whisk. You can opt for either a nonstick or a metal one. Using a whisk will ensure there aren't any clumps in your mixture.

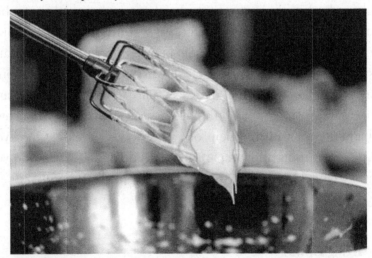

Measuring Cups

When you tackle the recipes, you will notice that you need to measure some of the ingredients before using them. A measuring cup will guarantee that you use the correct amount for the best results.

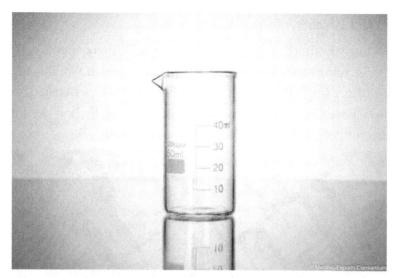

You probably already have a mixing bowl, a whisk, and a measuring cup in your kitchen, but if you don't, you can find them in Ikea, Amazon, or any store near you that sells cookware.

Rubber Gloves

You are going to mold the bath bombs with your hands, so a pair of rubber gloves will come in handy. In addition, using gloves is a lot more sanitary than using your bare hands. If you don't have any, you can easily find a large selection on Amazon.

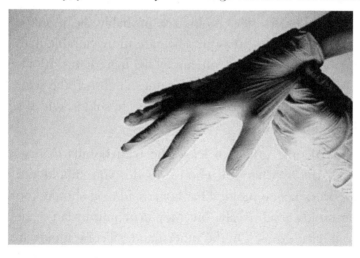

Paint Brush

After you finish making your bath bombs, there may be some powder residue left on the finished product, which you'll need to dust off. A small paintbrush will get the job done perfectly. If you don't have any paintbrushes at home, you'll find a huge collection on Amazon or your nearest DIY store.

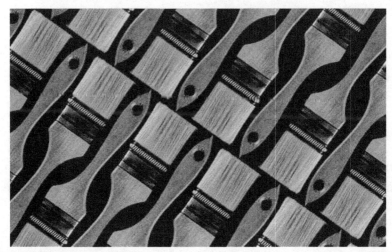

Bath Bombs Molds

Bath bomb molds are what give the bath bombs their unique and attractive shapes. They come in different shapes, sizes, and materials. Stainless steel molds are probably the most popular, and this is for a good reason. They are more durable than other materials and won't react with any of the ingredients. It's also very easy to clean stainless steel, and it doesn't absorb the scent from your essential oils. Stainless steel molds are sold in sets of six and come in different sizes.

Some people prefer to leave the bath bombs to dry in the mold. If this is what you choose to do, you should opt for a plastic or a silicone mold. That being said, you should know that plastic molds crack easily, but they do come in large packs, so you will have extras. On the other hand, silicone molds are a lot more functional and durable. Choosing a mold's size will depend on your bathtub. If you have a large bathtub, then you should opt for medium or large molds. Finding bath bomb molds is very easy as Amazon has a huge variety of shapes and sizes.

Don't worry if you can't find bath bomb molds or aren't keen on spending money on a new DIY project. There are other options. As a matter of fact, there are various items in your home that can work as molds like silicone cupcake cases, yogurt pots, Christmas decorations, shot glasses, ice cube trays, or chocolate molds. All of these options can serve as great bath bomb molds.

Coloring Your Bath Bombs

When you are shopping for bath bombs, you may find yourself drawn to one more than the other. What makes a bath bomb appealing is its color because the color is the first thing our eyes notice before we take in the shape or smell. Naturally, you want to give your homemade bath bombs equally beautiful and attractive colors. A word of caution here. We don't recommend using artificial colors at all because they contain chemicals. Remember that you are trying to make a natural and organic product that won't be harsh on your skin. Therefore, using chemicals will defeat the purpose of your DIY project.

Various natural methods can add beautiful colors to your bath bomb. Remember, your skin will absorb this product, so you should make sure that you use a colorant that won't cause any side effects. Plant-based powders are usually the best option because they won't cause a reaction to your skin or cause any health problems.

You can experiment with colors since there is a huge variety of options to work with. If you want pink bath bombs, then you should use a madder root powder. People who love blue-purple can opt for blueberry powder but if you want a pure purple color, then use Ratanjot powder. Turmeric powder will create a golden yellow color, while spirulina powder will make a blue-green color. You can use cocoa or coffee powder for brown, and for red bath bombs, Moroccan red clay is perfect. If you want more natural colors, you can use clay or fruit powders. Last but not least, you can also use food coloring since it is made of natural ingredients

Some people feel tempted to use more than one color. While there is nothing wrong with that, try to avoid similar colors or different shades of the same color until you are more experienced. However, if this is your first time, opt for one color first until you get the hang of it. Once you get used to the whole process, you can experiment with different colors. You can also make a rainbow-colored bath bomb by mixing blue, green, red, yellow, and orange together. Make sure that you use accurate measurements with the color you use so that every bath bomb is the exact color you want.

Hardening Bath Bombs

We use bath bombs to have a relaxing bath, and naturally, we want to savor the experience. For this reason, you want your bath bomb to last for as long as possible. The only way you can guarantee that is by hardening your bath bomb.

Be Careful with the Ingredients

We mentioned earlier that one of the most important tools you'll need is a measuring cup because you must use the right amount of each ingredient. If you use more than the recipe calls for, you will not get the results you are hoping for. For instance, if you aren't using the correct amount of liquid ingredients, you will end up with a soft bath bomb that breaks easily. Additionally, suppose the recipe specifies using water. In that case, it is preferable to substitute it with alcohol since it evaporates faster than water and won't retain any moisture, which can make the bath bomb crack.

The weather will also affect your mixtures. Suppose you live in an area with high humidity. In that case, you shouldn't overuse wet ingredients but opt for dry ingredients instead, like kaolin clay or cornstarch. Dry ingredients like cornstarch won't only harden the bath bombs but can also benefit your skin. Cornstarch soothes your skin, making it perfect for people who suffer from sunburns, itchiness, or skin allergies. Kaolin clay also soothes irritated skin and works as a natural cleanser, making it a perfect ingredient for bath bombs.

That being said, you shouldn't overdo it with the dry ingredients as they can make your bath bombs dry and easy to break, particularly if you are using any type of salts. If your bath bomb is too dry, then we recommend that you add more oils or witch hazel to give it moisture, so it won't crack. Witch hazel can be very beneficial to your skin as it also works on soothing it, as well as tightening pores, and preventing any skin damage.

Simply put, the key here is to balance wet and dry ingredients while also considering the humidity of the area that you're living in. Following the recipe is essential, but you can experiment with ingredients a little once you get the hang of things and understand how the weather and each ingredient interact and what affects the hardness of the bath bombs. With practice, you will become an expert in knowing which ingredients you should use and which to avoid. So, keep practicing until you get the desired results.

Basic Ingredients

While you will find many recipes that will help you create different bath bombs, there are some basic ingredients that you need to know about. They are stapled ingredients in every recipe. You should know that all of the ingredients mentioned in this book are all-natural, so they don't have any chemicals in them.

Citric Acid

Are you wondering how bath bombs make bubbles and foam? The secret is citric acid. It is what makes a bath bomb fizz. It is one of the most important ingredients. It is a natural ingredient that is usually found in citrus fruits. Citric acid is also the reason why your skin feels much smoother after using a bath bomb.

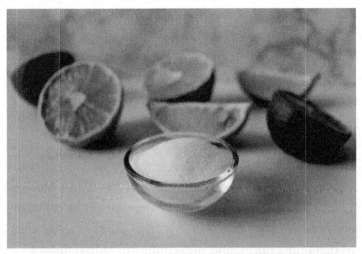

Baking Soda

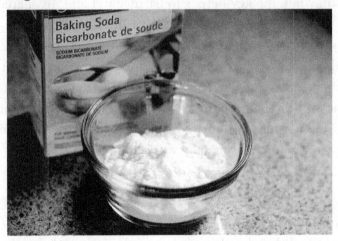

Baking soda, also called sodium bicarbonate, is considered one of the main ingredients because it works as a bonding agent. Baking soda is also a gentle exfoliant, and it is perfect for dry and rough skin because it can make the skin soft.

Essential Oils

Although essential oils are considered a basic ingredient, using them is optional. That being said, essential oils can be very beneficial to the skin as they can help with skin irritation, soothe

the skin, reduce wrinkles and any signs of aging of your skin. In addition to that, they make you feel relaxed, and they also smell gorgeous. However, some people don't like strong scents or are allergic to fragrances, so they opt out of using essential oils. There are various oils to choose from, like tea tree, lavender, or orange essential oils. You can use any essential oil you want as they can all work.

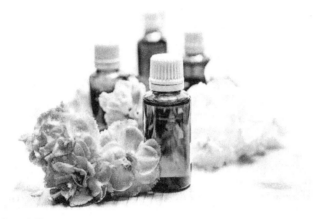

Carrier Oils

Carrier oils contain antioxidants and vitamins, which can give your skin a healthy and glowing look. There are different types of carrier oils to choose from, like sweet almond oil, avocado oil, olive oil, and coconut oil. Many people prefer coconut oil because it softens the skin. It is also considered one of the main ingredients because it works on holding the bath bomb together.

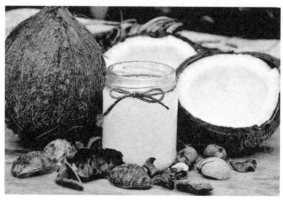

Witch Hazel

We have mentioned witch hazel and how it is one of the ingredients that can harden a bath bomb. Witch hazel is usually used instead of water or, in some circumstances, as a better option to water. This ingredient is plant-based, and it is perfect for soothing the skin.

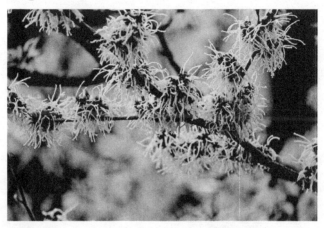

Epsom Salts

Some bath bomb ingredients soften and cleanse your skin, but Epsom salts have different benefits like soothing your sore muscles and relieving any muscle pain.

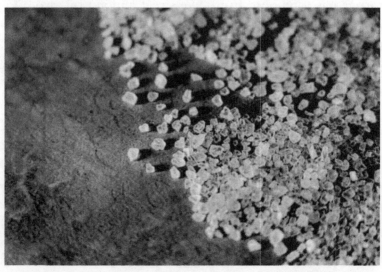

Cornstarch

Another ingredient that is essential for hardening the bath bomb is cornstarch. We have explained its benefits to your skin and for the bath bomb itself, which makes it an important ingredient.

Herbs

Whether dried or fresh, herbs can be very beneficial to your skin. Using herbs is optional, but many people use them because they are a great addition to the recipe and smell nice. There are many types of herbs to choose from. Some people opt for lavender for its lovely smell or chamomile for its soothing quality.

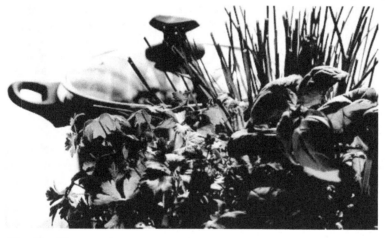

Kaolin Clay

As we have mentioned before, kaolin clay is an essential ingredient that will make your bath bomb harder than normal. It is gentle on the skin, and it cleanses and detoxes your skin.

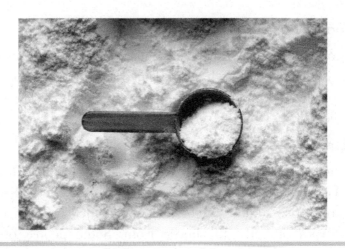

Decorative Ingredients

Decorative ingredients are ingredients that you can use to decorate your bath bombs. There are so many different ingredients that can make your bath bombs even more attractive, especially if you are going to give them away as gifts.

Glitter

Many girls love glitter. Glitter can be a great decoration for a bath bomb, especially if you have a little girl who loves to play with glitter or if you are planning to give it to someone as a gift. It will definitely make the bath bombs look more attractive. That being said, you should only use a small amount of glitter and make sure it's the eco-friendly kind.

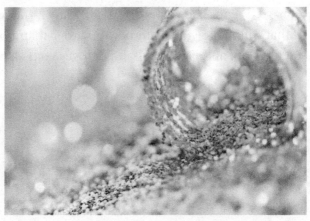

Sprinkles

If you are making a donut-shaped bath bomb, then you can decorate it with sprinkles to give it a realistic and delicious look. You can use regular food sprinkles as a decorative ingredient. They aren't toxic and will dissolve in the water immediately.

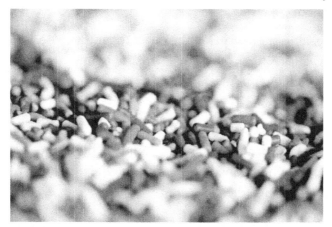

Dried Flowers

You can also use dried flowers to decorate your bath bomb. Put the dry petals in the bottom of the bath bomb mold before you place the mixture in the mold. When the bath bombs are done, the petals will be on top of them.

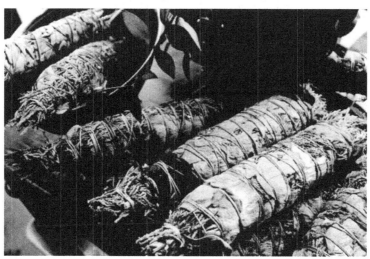

Ground Herbs

Just like dried flowers, put the ground herbs in the mold first, then add the mixture. As with the petals mentioned previously, the herbs will be on top of the bath bomb as well.

Bath Salt

Bath salt is another decorative ingredient that you can use. In order to make them stick to the bath bomb, you should use coconut oil. Don't use too much, though, or your bath bomb will not fizz.

There are two ways to add decorative ingredients; either to add them in with the other ingredients to be blended together, or, as we have mentioned, to put them in the mold before adding the mixture of ingredients.

Scent

If you want your bath bombs to smell lovely, then you should choose to use fragrance oils. There are so many to choose from – like vanilla, candy, pink sugar, and flowers. If you have kids, they will appreciate the nice aroma, especially cotton candy and ice cream. In addition to fragrance oils, you can also use perfume or vanilla essence. When it comes to the amount you will use, you can experiment a little. The quantity you add to your mix depends on the strength of scent you want in the end product. If you prefer more of a natural scent, you can use lavender, sandalwood, cinnamon, peppermint, or lemon.

Safety Notes

Practice makes perfect. However, if you are making something for the first time, then mistakes are bound to happen. For this reason, we want to give you a few safety notes and tips to put in mind while making your first batch.

Expanding Bath Bombs

While making your bath bombs, you may find that they expand. If this happens, don't fret, there is a solution. Expanding bath bombs is caused by a fizz reaction, and the cause is because you have probably added more water than recommended. You will have to add more citric acid or baking soda to remedy the situation.

Be Careful with Baking Soda

Baking soda causes skin irritations in some people. If this is the case for you, you should replace it with arrowroot powder.

Add Oils Slowly

Make sure that you do it slowly when you add oil to your mixture. The bath bomb may fizz in the mixing bowl if you add too much oil. Therefore, add the oils slowly so you won't accidentally add more than is required and ruin the recipe.

Allergies

Some people are allergic to perfumes and fragrances. If you have this type of allergy, don't use colorants or essential oils. You don't have to worry as they won't affect the recipe.

Making bath bombs at home is one of the easiest and most fun DIY projects out there. However, you will need to ensure you use the correct tools and ingredients to get the right results. Additionally, make sure you stick with the recipe, and once you figure everything out and get the hang of it, you will have the freedom to experiment with different ingredients. Last but not least, replace any ingredient that you are allergic to.

Chapter 3: What Essential Oils to Add

Essential oils are extracted from plants, and they usually have a very strong scent. They are also highly concentrated, which is why they shouldn't be applied directly to the skin. For this reason, carrier oils are used to dilute their concentration and make them safe for use. Essential oils are used in many skin products like shower gels, body lotions, and perfumes because of their popularity. The cosmetic industry incorporates them in many of their products because they have so many benefits for the skin. Some benefits of essential oils include reducing stretch marks, scars, wrinkles, itchiness, and soothing the skin.

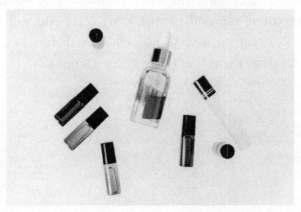

Essential oils are considered natural products, which is why many people use them when making organic bath bombs. Additionally, they will also give your bath bombs a natural fragrance. There are a lot of chemicals used in making commercial bath bombs that can penetrate the skin, which has led to many people making their own organic and natural products at home to avoid the use of chemicals. If you look at the list of ingredients on some of the commercial bath bombs, you will find a few you have probably never heard of before. For this reason, choosing a non-toxic and natural product is a safer option all around.

Benefits of Adding Essential Oils to Your Bath Bomb Recipe

Safe to Use

Essential oils are natural products extracted from plants, so they are safe to use, unlike other chemicals used in making commercial bath bombs. Remember that the ingredients you use in your bath bombs will penetrate your skin as you soak in luxury, so using natural essential oils will ensure there are no toxins in your carefully crafted works of art.

Reduce Wrinkles

The signs of aging usually show on the skin first, whether in wrinkles or fine lines. Essential oils can reduce the signs of aging and make your skin look fresh. The oils work on tightening the skin, reducing wrinkles and giving you a youthful look. You can add any type of essential oil; for example, lemon or orange oils are particularly beneficial to anti-aging, leaving your skin looking younger.

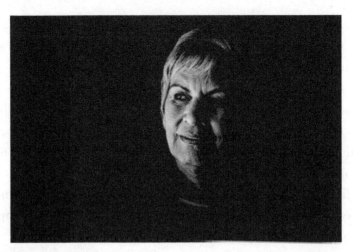

To Reduce Scars

There is no denying that we all wish for perfect-looking skin. Stretch marks, scars, and sun damage are some of the skin flaws that we all want to get rid of. One of the natural products that can help with these skin issues is essential oils because they contain herbs and natural ingredients that can be very beneficial to the skin.

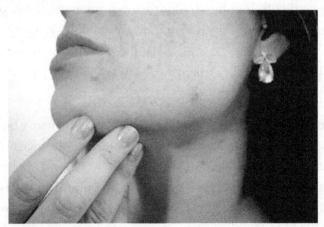

Calming Effect

These oils are great to help your mind, body, and skin relax and de-stress. Essential oils like lemon oil, lavender oil, or orange oil are ideal for helping you get rid of the day's worries because these scents are the best for calming and helping you unwind.

Reduces Irritation

Many people suffer from skin irritation for different reasons, like itches and rashes. Suppose you are constantly suffering from irritated skin. In that case, you can try adding tea tree oil or peppermint oil (known for its cooling effect) to your bath bomb ingredients.

Enhances the Skin

Severe weather conditions can seriously impact our skin and change its texture. Citrus essential oils like lemon or orange oil can help enhance the skin's texture and make it look radiant and fresh.

Provide Stress Relief

There is no denying that stress has become a serious problem that many people suffer from. One of the most popular relaxation methods is taking a long, warm bath. Essential oils are known for promoting relaxation and stress relief. Therefore, adding essential oils like lavender, lemongrass, lemon, or orange to your bath bomb recipe will contribute to relieving your stress. Additionally, the scents of essential oils can calm your mind, which can really help people suffering from anxiety.

Improves Sleep

People who have trouble falling asleep usually take a warm bath to help them sleep better. The scent of essential oil like lavender can help improve your sleep. So, adding it to your bath bomb recipe and taking a bath before bed will make you fall asleep faster in a wonderfully natural way.

Side Effects of Essential Oils

Using essential oils diluted in a carrier oil for a skin product is pretty safe. That being said, nothing is perfect, and although essential oils have many benefits, they can have side effects as well. In some cases, essential oils can cause rashes, headaches, asthma, and allergies. In order to be safe, make sure that the essential oils you are going to use are diluted with carrier oils to reduce their concentration. Generally, diluted essential oils are considered safe.

However, suppose you suffer from any of those conditions. In that case, there are some essential oils that you should steer clear of, for example, thyme, oregano, black pepper, clove, camphor, wintergreen, and spearmint.

Essential Oils for Bath Bombs

After understanding the pros and cons of using these oils, adding them to your list of ingredients seems like a good idea. Because there is such a wide variety of oils to choose from, we have looked in more depth at a few of the more commonly used oils.

Chamomile Oil

You've probably heard about the benefits of chamomile tea and how it is usually recommended for people who need to calm down or fall asleep. Chamomile oil has a similar effect on your body and skin. This oil can soothe the skin, reduce inflammation, defend the skin against wrinkles, calm irritations and rashes, and hydrate and moisturize the skin. In addition, it promotes relaxation, reduces anxiety, and helps you sleep better.

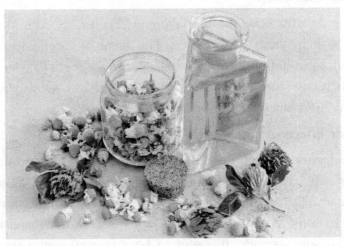

If you are allergic to chamomile or any ragweed plant, then you should steer clear of chamomile oil. However, if you aren't sure if you are allergic, test it by putting a drop of the diluted oil on the inside of your elbow. People with a chamomile allergy will feel and see their skin get itchy, red, or burning.

In combination with lavender, Chamomile smells wonderful and serves up a double dose of relaxation-promoting properties. This is a really good demonstration of how using more than one oil works just as well, if not even better, in your bath bomb recipe.

Lavender Oil

As we have just explained, lavender oil, like chamomile oil, is really great for soothing the skin. It's a popular ingredient to use in your bath bomb because, in addition to being a relaxant, it is also very useful for detoxifying the skin and releasing any tension in your muscles, leaving you smelling good and completely relaxed. Besides relaxation, lavender oil also calms your skin and mind. It reduces stress and anxiety and soothes irritated skin as well. Lavender oil also has a gentle fragrance that will give your bath bomb a softly fragrant scent.

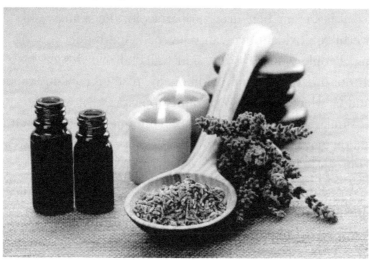

For the most part, lavender oil doesn't have any side effects when applied to the skin. However, if you have any allergies to the plant, then you could suffer from skin irritation which is why a test is important.

Tea Tree Oil

You have probably heard about tea tree oil, and if you have oily skin, then you've probably used it. Tea tree oil reduces acne and acne scars as it removes oil from the skin's surface. It also fights inflammation which helps to reduce itchiness and redness in your skin. Tea tree oil will also make your skin look clear and smooth. People suffering from dry skin can also benefit from this oil since it moisturizes and soothes dry skin. Another condition it is good for is to reduce dark spots on your body. Unlike some oily skin products, tea tree oil doesn't cause any dryness to your skin. However, we recommend it not be used at all if you're suffering from hormone-dependent cancer or are pregnant.

Rose Oil

It goes without saying that rose oil smells good. So, if you are a fan of flowery fragrances, then you shouldn't hesitate about adding rose oil to your bath bomb. Besides its nice fragrance, rose oil has many beneficial properties for the skin as well. It's a powerful antioxidant that can rejuvenate and reduce any signs of aging. People who have dry skin will find that this oil hydrates and moisturizes the skin. Additionally, rose oil contains vitamins A and C, which can slow down the appearance of wrinkles. Rose oil, similar to Lavender and Chamomile oil, also reduces irritation and redness and soothes it thanks to its anti-inflammatory qualities.

You should know that undiluted rose oil isn't safe for pregnant women and may cause miscarriage.

Cedarwood Oil

Cedarwood oil may not be as popular and well known as some of the names we've already mentioned, but it is still equally useful. Cedarwood oil is extracted from the cedar tree. It's a pleasant-smelling oil that can calm your mind, reduce anxiety, and help you sleep better. It also soothes and reduces acne, itching, and inflammation. The scent of cedarwood oil has a calming effect on people suffering from depression, stress, or anxiety. Cedar oil is also safe and doesn't have any side effects, so you can add it to your recipe without any worry.

Ylang-Ylang Oil

Ylang-ylang oil is extracted from a flower found in Asian countries like the Philippines and Indonesia. The fragrant oil promotes relaxation and helps to reduce anger, stress, and anxiety. Ylang-ylang can be used by people who have oily skin because it helps to reduce acne. It is also an anti-aging aid, reducing the signs of aging like wrinkles and fine lines. It is also a moisturizer and rejuvenates the skin, making it the perfect ingredient for people with dry skin. Bonus properties are that it has a sedative effect and can lower heart rate and blood pressure.

People suffering from anxiety should use ylang-ylang oil with rose oil to calm their nerves. Since ylang-ylang can help lower blood pressure and rose oil can help with depression, adding both oils to your bath bomb can positively impact your mental health.

A word of caution – ylang-ylang may cause an allergic reaction. However, this only happens if it is applied directly to the skin. Remember, we have mentioned that essential oils should never be directly applied to the skin.

Turmeric Oil

Turmeric oil is extracted from a plant by the same name and makes a great addition to your stock of ingredients because of its effect on acne. It can reduce and dry out acne and blemishes, leaving your skin looking fresh and clear. Turmeric oil can also be a great solution for people who have dull-looking skin as it rejuvenates while also reducing inflammation and wrinkles to make you look younger. Turmeric oil has also been known to relieve symptoms of depression.

Turmeric oil is safe since it doesn't have any side effects.

Lemongrass Oil

Lemongrass oil has a very light, clean, and refreshing scent, making it an ideal ingredient for bath bombs. Something else that makes it a great ingredient is that it is a powerful cleanser, which is why it is used in products like soaps, shampoos, and bath bombs. Using lemongrass oil will leave your skin fresh and glowing. Lemongrass oil's scent helps reduce anxiety, is calming, and helps you to feel calm and less irritable. Therefore, taking a bath in your new lemongrass bath bombs after a long and stressful day at work will definitely relax and calm your nerves. A lemongrass bath bomb is a great way to start the day, feeling fresh and energetic. Although lemongrass is safe when applied to the skin, in some cases, it has been known to cause toxic side effects. This is why skin tests are essential.

Eucalyptus Oil

Eucalyptus Oil is extracted from the leaves of eucalyptus trees native to Australia. This oil has a wide range of beneficial properties, such as reducing pain and relieving tight muscles. Additionally, it soothes the skin, reduces redness, acne, and treats sunburns. Eucalyptus oil can also improve your mood, calm your mind, reduce stress, and make you feel refreshed.

Although eucalyptus oil can benefit your skin and mental health, its safety isn't guaranteed even if diluted.

Frankincense Oil

Frankincense oil has been used ever since the time of the Ancient Egyptians, who considered it a holy oil. It is extracted from a tree called Boswellia in Africa. This oil is an antioxidant which means that it can slow down the signs of aging. It also moisturizes the skin, protects it from dryness, soothes inflammation, reduces acne, and protects the skin from damage.

Frankincense oil doesn't have any side effects and has been used safely for years now.

We can't stress enough how important it is to only use diluted essential oils. Essential oils shouldn't be applied to the skin undiluted, or they can cause severe irritations and burns. Although almost all of the oils that we've listed here are considered safe, they may not be safe for you. So as a good cautionary practice, test every essential oil on your skin first before using it in your bath bombs.

Testing the oil is very easy. You will need to apply one or two drops of diluted oil to your inner elbow or wrist. If you start to itch, then this means that you are allergic to the oil and that you shouldn't use it or even touch it again. If you don't display any reaction, you should test it one more time just to be safe.

If you're pregnant or breastfeeding, it isn't recommended to use essential oils during these critical times. However, if you must use them, you should speak with your doctor first.

Some recipes won't specify which essential oil you should use. In this case, you can choose any oil you want, and you can always experiment with them. It is also important to note that you should only add five drops of the oil unless the recipe specifies a different quantity.

How to Use Essential Oils with Kids

Bath time for kids will change forever when you start using bath bombs. The color and bubbles will make bathing a really fun experience. You will battle to get the kids out of the bath. However, you can't use the exact same size bomb for kids as you can with adults. Below we have outlined the safe-use quantities for each age group.

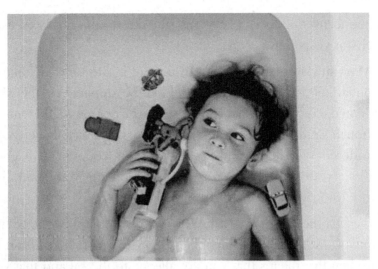

One Year Or Less

If you have a newborn baby or a baby that is one year or less, then you should only use one drop. That being said, you can't use just any kind of essential oil. For instance, some oils won't be safe for babies, like peppermint, eucalyptus, and rosemary oil. However, essential oils like chamomile or lavender are good choices for babies at this age.

Two to Five Years Old

You can increase the dosage a little for kids from two years old to five years old. You can use three drops of essential oils. You should still avoid the oils that we've mentioned above because they can cause breathing problems. Stick to the soothing oils, like lavender and chamomile. And be mindful that their skin is extremely delicate at this age, so don't use oils that penetrate the skin.

Five to Twelve Years Old

Now that your children are growing, you can use half the amount specified in the bath bomb recipe. For instance, if the recipe specifies that you use six drops, you should only use three drops.

Remember to dilute the essential oils with carrier oils before using them. It's also recommended to ask your doctor first before using essential oils on your kids or if you are pregnant or breastfeeding. Essential oils have so many benefits, and naturally, you want to take advantage of them and add them to your homemade bath bond recipe. However, caution is key here. You have to make sure that the oils are safe and that you aren't allergic to any of them. Test each oil you plan to add using the method we have mentioned above. Last but not least, you should know that essential oils should never be consumed. For this reason, keep your bottles of essential oils away from your children and pets.

Chapter 4: Basic Bath Bomb Recipe and Customization

Apart from being of great use in anyone's skincare routine, bath bombs can be a fun experiment. Homemade bath bombs are made of natural ingredients – which are generally perfectly safe to handle and use on the skin. With a little bit of practice and creativity, you can craft personalized products for yourself or anyone else if they are going to be a gift. However, before experimenting with the ingredients, it's good to learn how bath bombs actually work. This chapter will help you understand the main components of bath bombs. It also contains a comprehensive scientific explanation of the purpose of each main element, along with a few tips on how to adjust them if needed. Lastly, you will be advised on possible customization techniques and ingredients that can take your bath bomb-making skills to a whole new level.

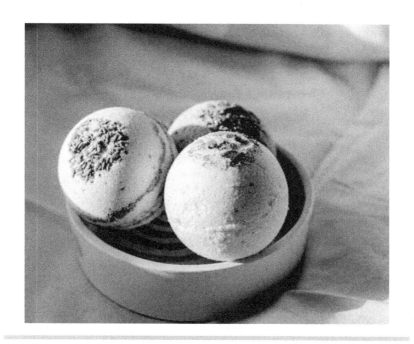

Bath Bomb Ingredients

Depending on who you're making them for, bath bombs can consist of a wide variety of ingredients, from fragrant oils (especially for relaxation) to oils that can soothe and soften sore muscles and calm an anxious, stressed body at the end day.

And when you are crafting a bath bomb at home, you can choose to add any ingredient you like. However, for these additions to work their magnificent powers on you, you must get the basic ingredients put together correctly, and they are – citric acid, baking soda, and cornstarch. Each of these elements has a specific role in a bath bomb, and without them, you won't be able to create an effective product. In fact, they are present in most store-bought bath bombs as well, along with a myriad of other ingredients – many of which are unnecessary.

When combined, citric acid and baking soda create that fizzing and bubbling effect that makes using bath bombs so enjoyable. If you are wondering how they do that – well, the explanation is pretty simple. It all comes down to a chemical reaction between an acid, a base, and a stabilizing agent. Citric acid is a weak acid, while baking soda is a mild base, and both of them are activated in the water. So, when you combine them in a bath bomb which you then place in the water, they will begin to dissolve. This triggers the reaction between them, which results in the release of CO2 (carbon dioxide). CO2 is a gas that makes the fizzing and the bubbling you see. However, combining only citric acid and baking soda will result in a very abrupt reaction, which means that you end up with a bath bomb that fizzles out in seconds. The binding properties of cornstarch slow down the reaction between acid and base, so you can have a pleasurable bubbling experience that lasts for a couple of minutes.

Basic Bath Bomb Recipe

This basic bath bomb recipe uses the three main ingredients, citric acid, baking soda, and cornstarch, along with binding agents. Here, vegetable oil and water are used for this purpose, but the recipe can be amended to fit individual needs. The addition of oil creates a mild formula suitable for every skin type, while the reactive agents provide a pleasantly relaxing bathing experience.

Ingredients

- Citric acid - 1/3 cup or 50g
- Baking soda - 1/2 cup or 115g
- Cornstarch - 1/5 cup or 25g
- Vegetable oil - 2 tbsp or 30 ml
- Water - as needed

Other Equipment You Will Need

- Measuring spoons
- Utensils for mixing
- Mixing bowls

- An ice cube tray, muffin tray, or bath bomb molds

- Pastry brush – optional

- Medicine dropper – optional

Where to Find the Ingredients

Citric acid is often used in winemaking, candies, and homemade canned products, and you'll find it in the grocery aisle of any supermarket. Baking soda and cornstarch are essential pantry ingredients, usually available at your local convenience store. If you decide to spruce up your bath bombs with other ingredients – like food coloring or essential oils – you can buy these in pharmacies and supermarkets, as well.

Directions

1. Put citric acid, baking soda, and cornstarch in a large bowl, and mix them until well combined. If you are adding an optional dry ingredient, you may incorporate that at this stage.

2. Start adding the vegetable oil to the dry ingredients. You must do this slowly because the reactive ingredients will start interacting as soon as they contact the wet ones; this is where your medicine dropper comes in handy to make sure you control the addition of wet ingredients to the dry ones.

3. If you notice that the mixture starts fizzing in any place, press down on the fizz with the back of a spoon, then quickly mix the wet spot into the rest of the mixture. Make sure the sizzling stops before you add more moisture.

4. Repeat the process until you've added all the oil. Your mixture should be moist enough to be molded in your hand without crumbling or dripping out of your hands. Make sure you check this now because the consistency of the wet mixture can affect the end product.

5. If it's too dry – and it crumbles in your hands – you may add a few drops of water, and if it's too wet, you can soak up the excess moisture by adding a little bit more cornstarch.

6. Once all your ingredients are thoroughly mixed – and you're with the "moldability" of your formula – it's now ready to be put into your molds.

7. Coat your mold or tray with a little oil, spreading it with your fingers or a pastry brush. Then fill the molds by scooping it one spoonful at a time. Make sure you press each scoop down with the back of the spoon.

8. After filling your molds evenly, you then dry your bath bombs. If your environment is on the drier side, you may leave them to dry uncovered at room temperature overnight. If the environment is humid, it's recommended to dry the bath bombs in a preheated oven at 170°F (or approximately 75°C – which is typically the lowest setting) for 45 minutes.

9. You can check the dryness of your bath bombs by tapping them with your fingers or the back of a spoon. Their surface should feel hard and solid. Once dry, remove the bath bombs from the molds.

10. And there you have it! Perfectly homemade bath bombs ready for immediate use. If you're not going to use them straight away, they can be stored in an airtight container in a dry and cool place for several weeks.

This recipe can fill three average-sized ice cube cups or one larger muffin cup. However, if you are using any other molds or sizing, you will probably get different proportions. If you want to make more, adjust the amounts accordingly. When doing so, just make sure you double or triple all the ingredients proportionally to get a proper formula. If you are making bath bombs for the first time, it is recommended to dry them and try them out in warm water right away. This way, you'll find out if you need to make any adjustments to the formula or not.

Tips and Tricks for Bath Bomb Customization

The most challenging part of making a bath bomb for beginners is getting the number of wet ingredients right. Remember, we have already spoken about your weather and how it affects moisture levels and the temperature of your environment. For example, if you live in a drier climate or are making bath bombs in a warm, heating kitchen, you will need to add more wet ingredients to your formula. You may find that even after combining all components, the mixture still crumbles out of your hands. Or you may have the opposite problem – your bath bombs keep swelling up after mixing, which means they probably have too much moisture in them. As mentioned in the directions, you can adjust the moisture levels of your mixture with a little bit of cornstarch or water before completing the mixing process. However, you will only be able to do this while the bath bombs are still moist. Once they dry completely, the only way to fix them is to make a new batch.

If you aren't sure if the mixture will hold up when dried, you can make two batches at once, one with a little less cornstarch and one with a little more. Cornstarch slows down the rate of the reaction between the other two ingredients. By changing the amount, you affect the fizziness of your bath bombs. For example, if you want to make a bath bomb that fizzles out slower, you can do this by simply increasing the amount of cornstarch in the mixture. Keep in mind this will make the formula drier, so you'll have to compensate with water or some other wet ingredient. If you find that your formula works better with less moisture, adjust the recipe for the next batch. As long as you are doing it in the same conditions (humidity and temperature-wise), you should have no problems making the perfect bath bombs.

Another stabilizer you can use is Kaolin clay, which adds an extra dimension to your bomb as well as being a stabilizer. Add ½ tsp of Kaolin clay to the dry ingredients before mixing them with the wet ones. The clay will bond with vegetable oil, so your bombs will harden up quicker and dissolve slower, as well as add its soothing properties.

On the other hand, if you want to create more bubbles and fizzle in your bathwater, you can simply increase the amount of baking soda and citric acid used in the mixture. Pay attention to the proportions - it should always be one part of citric acid and two parts baking soda. You can even try a batch entirely without cornstarch. And, if you feel the "dough" is too wet, you may add other dry ingredients, such as dried herbs. They will soak up the moisture without interfering with the acid-base reaction. However, this will make your bath bomb dissolve quicker - but you will be able to enjoy the other beneficial effects of its ingredients longer.

If you want to test how long it takes for a bomb to dissolve, you can try out your bath bombs right away, but make sure to do it in warm water. Cold water also slows down the acid-base reaction time, but you won't know how your ingredients will react in an actual hot water bath. By the same token, you shouldn't put them in scalding hot water either because this will cause a very intense reaction. The same is true when you use your bombs in your bath - have your water moderately hot, and they will bubble for much longer, not to mention that avoiding baths with overly hot water is also healthier for you.

When it comes to molds, remember that the size of your finished product will have an effect on how long they last in a bath. The larger you make your bath bombs, the longer it will take them to dissolve. So, if you want to enjoy your bubbles as long as you can, it's a good idea to look for a mold that will give you the biggest bombs possible. Or, if you are making spheres or any other particular shapes, an even better solution is to make smaller halves and stick them together with a little bit of water once dried. This will cut down the drying time, and you'll have nicely shaped bath bombs. Just make sure the mold you're using is flexible enough - so you don't crush the dried product when removing the bombs from the mold. And don't forget to oil your mold before putting the wet mixture in either, particularly if you aren't using silicone molding.

Another tip - when putting out the small fizzing spot during the mixing process, dry your spoon before touching the mixture. Avoid touching the dry ingredients with anything. If you are making several batches, use separate tools for each one of them to make sure they are clean and dry. Even if you aren't using coloring, you may still end up using wet ones, in which case you will have a lot of unnecessary acid-base reactions to deal with, and you may have to start the process all over again. The more cornstarch you add to the mixture, the less likely this will happen, whereas if you use little or no filler, the more fizzling you'll get even during the mixing process. Another solution to avoid this is to add citric acid after mixing all the other ingredients together. While this can make things harder to combine, it can delay the reaction, which means you will get more bubbles and fizzle in the bathtub.

If you're adding wet ingredients, this also means that you will have to adjust the amounts of the primary ones. For example, if you are using liquid food coloring and essential oils, you probably won't need to add any water. In fact, you may need to reduce the amount of vegetable oil or increase the amount of cornstarch in the recipe. Adding less or no water to your mixture comes with a couple of advantages. For one, if you are using any food coloring, they won't get diluted and will stay vivid even when you dissolve your bath bombs in water. As a plus, without water, you won't get as much reaction during the preparation. You will work faster and more efficiently, which is always better when making bath bombs. The sooner you can get them into the mold, the sooner they will begin to dry, and less chance the citric acid and the baking soda will have to interact with each other.

Provided you keep them in a dry and cool environment, your bath bombs will stay intact for longer. The amount and the quality of wet ingredients affect the drying time; for example, water evaporates faster, so if you are drying your batch at room temperatures, more water-based formulas will definitely dry in a couple of hours. However, oils will take much longer to dry, so if you are substituting water with oil-based products, you will have to leave your bath bombs to dry for 24-48 hours. You want to make sure they are completely dry before storing them away. Keep them away from moisture when storing because even humidity can set them off. So, an airtight container is the best storage option, from humidity as well as to preserve any fragrance you've used. Adjusting your main ingredients to get the perfect bath bomb consistency is not the only way to customize the basic recipe. You can also do it by adding components to suit the needs of individual skin types. Here are some ideas on what you can add to your bath bombs.

Some of the most popular additional ingredients for bath bombs are:

- Food coloring

- Epsom salts

- Essential oils

- Dried herbs

- Citrus peels

When it comes to food coloring, avoid using gels. Despite providing a more vivid color in baked products, they can't be combined with baking soda. As soon as these two ingredients come into contact, the gel begins to clump, and it will be impossible to mix it well. For this reason, only use liquid food coloring. There are many ways to spruce these up, as well –

mixing several colors, making a rainbow bath bomb, or layering colors are only some of the ways to do so. Reducing the amount of wet ingredients used may also result in more vibrantly colored bath bombs. Feel free to experiment with the amount of coloring you use by adding one drop at a time.

Of course, using essential oils makes your bath bombs smell lovely – as we discussed in previous chapters, and they add all sorts of healing, self-care properties to your bath experience. Be careful with the amounts you use, as some of them are very potent, and even a few drops will be enough of them. The most you will need is about 15-20 drops, even from the more delicately scented oils. Use a medicine dropper when working with such small quantities as this will help to ensure you don't go overboard. If you're using several essential oils, make sure the medicine dropper is clean before using it for each oil. If you want a less intense fragrance, you may use dried herbs, like rose petals or crushed lavender leaves in your mixture as well. These herbs are also decorative and can make your bombs look delightful, especially when you're making them as gifts.

Another way to customize your bath bombs is by adding salts to them. One of the most popular salts used in bath bombs is Epsom salt - which, besides being a very effective exfoliant, also has antiseptic properties. Soaking in salts is often beneficial for sensitive and problematic skin. While the main ingredients are essential for making the bath bombs effective, in some cases, even those ingredients can be substituted. For example, if you are unable to find the citric acid or prefer not to use it, you can switch it up with citrus juice or tartaric acid. Citrus juice adds a particularly invigorating quality to your bath bombs, plus it can even act as a gentle exfoliator during your bath. Likewise, citrus peels also have the same effect on the skin but without affecting the acidity of your mixture.

Chapter 5: Bath Bombs for Kids

With endless chores, work duties, homework, technology, screen time, and the other overly consuming aspects of life, it becomes harder and harder to spend quality time with our families. The lack of family time not only weakens the bond that we have with our parents, siblings, spouse, or children, but it also takes a negative toll on our physical, mental, and spiritual well-being. Having a family is a blessing, and kids make you feel happy and fulfilled. According to Highland Springs, a specialty clinic, several studies have shown that spending time with family helps diminish the symptoms of anxiety and stress. Healthy families make each member feel valued and motivated. They help each other reach their full potential and unlock the best version of themselves. The best way to revitalize family relationships and foster a healthy connection is by making something together as a family, and making bath bombs with your kids is the perfect way to do so.

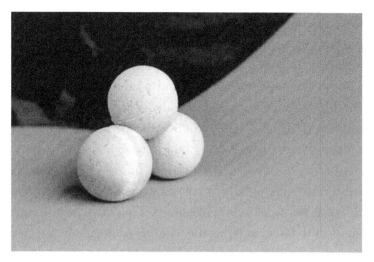

Making bath bombs together helps to enhance their focus, academic performance, and self-confidence. And, because it comprises several precise steps and procedures, making bath bombs with your kids has some amazing spin-offs in terms of your kid's development. The process and ingredients are tricky enough for an adult to get right, so if your child can do it, you are boosting their confidence, trust, creativity, and patience skills, which will also spill over into the way they work at school. Creating a bath bomb can be an exciting process, which is why your kids will be keen on getting all the steps right. This will teach them the importance of staying dedicated and focused on one task.

Making a bath bomb with your child allows them to explore their creativity, skills, and abilities. It also helps reinforce positive behaviors and serves as an outlet for repressed emotions. Instead of spending their time glued to a screen, they will be honing their math, learning science in real life, and being creative, and – the cherry on the top is a really fun bath time. Since making bath bombs is generally a new idea, it allows them to take a break from the boring routine and encourages them to think out of the box. Trying out new things with your kids is likely to make them less afraid of challenges and new things.

As you may have noticed, this family activity is so much more than throwing a few ingredients together. In addition to the numerous benefits for your child and family members, creating a bath bomb has both a scientific and a crafting facet. It requires you to follow a recipe, play around with the ingredients and consistencies, as well as explore the possibility of entirely customizing your own. Your child gets to explore quite a few different areas of interest. Even if their hobby doesn't turn out to be bath bomb-making, they may discover their love for following recipes or even tweaking them a little. They may find themselves intrigued and fascinated by the chemistry angle of the activity. You never know, but your child may become the next world-famous chemist or Michelin, Starred chef.

Now that you know how making bath bombs can be rewarding for the entire family, read on to discover numerous bath bomb recipes for children. Each recipe is rated for its level of difficulty and includes thorough instructions on how you can make them.

Why Your Kid Should Use DIY Bath Bombs

Before you go through the recipes, you need to read up on why your kid needs to use bath bombs. For some reason, when we hear the words "bath bomb," our minds immediately wander to candles, essential oils, wine, and soft music. We picture an adult preparing their bath to unwind from a stressful day at work. It's not often that you come across bath bombs particularly made for children, even though they'll be overjoyed just by watching it dissolve into the bath, changing the color of the water. They'll be excited to hop into the tub and surround themselves with the colorful foam. Bath bombs have so much more to offer than just their aesthetic. They can be equally beneficial for adults and children alike.

Bath time becomes a lot easier and way more fun when you have a bath bomb. If you're a parent, you know the struggle of getting your kids to take a bath. Children will do anything to get out of it. They may try to convince you that they're hurt or have even suddenly developed a soap allergy out of nowhere to avoid bathing. You may have to run around the house a couple of times, shout, cajole, threaten to ground them, and even bribe them with a post-bath treat before you finally get them to agree to get their hygiene fix for the day. It's not easy to go through the same tiring routine every day. Unfortunately, bath time, which is supposed to be associated with positive things, becomes dreadful for you and your child. Having a bath bomb, however, can turn things around. The chances are that your child will go from despising baths to looking forward to bath time if you allow them to use a bath bomb. They'd be even more excited if they've made it themselves since they'd be curious to find out if they made it work. Some children's bath bombs even dissolve to reveal a surprise toy inside, which is a huge plus.

Bath bombs are generally safe for children aged three and above. This is because children typically do not develop strong enough skin until they're three years old. Either way, it's best if you conduct a patch test on your child to make sure that they're not allergic to any of the ingredients. You should also make sure to rinse your child off well after the bath to get rid of any residue. Even if they're not allergic, their skin may become irritated if the ingredients are left on for too long.

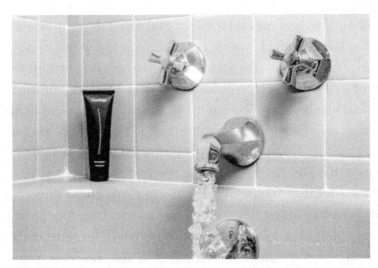

Children's skin is a lot more sensitive than adults'. This is because they have a less thick and less tight outer layer of skin. Their sweat glands are not as active either. Their skin also lacks protective natural oils or fats. This all makes them more likely to develop eczema, skin rashes, and other skin conditions triggered by harsh chemicals. This is why you should refrain from using store-bought bath bombs, even if the label claims that it's all-natural. The only way to be sure the product is safe and made from entirely natural ingredients is when you've made it yourself.

Many bath bombs that are advertised as organic or safe include SLES, which is an ingredient otherwise known as sodium laurate sulfate. SLES is a skin irritant and may be especially harmful to individuals with prior skin conditions like psoriasis and eczema, and of course, children with sensitive skin. Companies love to add this ingredient because it provides extra foaming, which makes the bath bomb more appealing. It doesn't really add to the effectiveness of the product.

You can make amazing bath bombs at home using moisturizing and natural ingredients, such as apricot kernels, almonds, jojoba, and coconut oils. You won't have to worry about ingredients like parabens and SLES. Homemade bath bombs also serve as a wonderful alternative to bubble baths.

Regular soaps and shower gels are also often loaded with harsh fragrances and chemicals, which could lead to infections in the urinary tract in children. The soapy residue left by commercial products is often difficult to wash off and may irritate sensitive skin. Fortunately, natural oils and ingredients found in bath bombs don't cause these kinds of infections.

Things to Keep in Mind

As we've mentioned, bath bombs are only safe for children if they're made of natural materials. This is why you should avoid bath bombs that include flavorings and fragrances used to enhance the smell of essential oils, artificial dyes, glitters, and of course, parabens and SLES. You should also look out for the expiration dates. You need to keep in mind that you won't be using chemically-curated preservatives if you're making your own bath bombs.

Before allowing your kid to use the product, consider their age in relation to their skin development, as we previously explained. You should also be mindful of how frequently you bathe them with bath bombs. Although your child may expect to use one every time they get in the bathtub, you need to make it clear that they won't be able to use them every day. Even though DIY products are free of chemicals, natural ingredients can become irritating when used excessively.

DIY Bath Bombs

All homemade bath bombs are generally formulated using the same base. The best thing about bath bombs is that their simple formula makes them very easy to make and leaves plenty of room for creativity. You get to choose which essential oils to use and how you want to scent and color your base.

The standard ingredients used to make the base of just about any bath bomb are:

- Baking powder- 1 cup or 128g

- Epsom salts- 1/2 cup or 64g

- Citric acid- 1/2 cup or 64g

- Corn starch- 1/2 cup or 64g

However, the exact quantities may differ according to the type of bath bomb you'll be making. While you can use this base to experiment with your own ideas, the following are a few recipes or formulations that you can try out for kids. Each of them comes with a scale rating its level of difficulty (one being the lowest and five the highest), so you can choose one that suits you and your child.

Soothing Bath Bomb★☆☆☆☆

This bath bomb has quite a few steps to it and is a bomb with soothing properties that will help soften your child's skin. This formula will help your child feel relaxed and get a good night's sleep.

Ingredients

- Baking powder- 1 cup or 128g

- Citric acid- 1/3 cup or 32g (the deviation from the standard recipe makes the bath bomb milder)

- Corn starch- 3 tbsps

- Melted coconut oil- 1 tbsp

- Your choice of food coloring- 4 to 8 drops (the number of drops depends on the shade you're aiming for).

- Lavender essential oil- 10 drops

- Oatmeal colloidal powder- 1/2 cup or 64g

Where to Find the Ingredients

You'll find these ingredients at any convenience store, aromatherapists, and organic shops.

Directions

- Mix the cornstarch and the baking powder in a large bowl.

- Add the food coloring to your desired color, along with a few drops of warm water. Make sure you mix them really well.

- In a separate bowl, mix all your oils together. Mix well, then add it to the bowl with the dry ingredients.

- Use your hands or a whisk to blend them together well.

- Finally, add your citric acid and make sure that the formula feels like wet sand.

- Allow it to sit for a few minutes in a bomb mold.

Tips and Tricks:

- Make sure not to use too much warm water as it can mess with the consistency of the mixture.

Substitutes:

- You can switch the oatmeal colloidal powder with Epsom salts. The oatmeal colloidal powder is a softer exfoliant that nourishes the skin.

Citrusy Cupcake ★★☆☆☆

This bath bomb is very easy to make, and its scent doesn't fall short of the smell of cupcakes. Its citrusy notes will leave your child feeling fresh and energized.

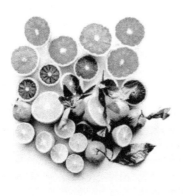

Ingredients

- Baking powder- 1 cup or 128g

- Epsom salts- 1/2 cup or 64g

- Citric acid- 1/2 cup or 64g

- Corn starch- 1/2 cup or 64g

- Coconut oil- 4 tbsps

- Bergamot grapefruit essential oil- 10 drops (you can also use any other citrusy essential oil of your choice).

- Pink food coloring- 4 to 8 drops (the number of drops depends on the shade you're aiming for).

- Vanilla essential oil- 10 drops

Where to Find the Ingredients

You can get your hands on any of these ingredients at any convenience store. For high-quality essential oils and coconut oil, you can check out organic shops or specialized aromatherapy retailers.

Directions

1. Pour your baking powder, Epsom salts, and cornstarch into a large mixing bowl. Stir the ingredients well to mix them together.

2. Grab a microwave-safe bowl or measuring cup and add your coconut oil, food coloring, Bergamot grapefruit essential oil (or your choice of scent), as well as a vanilla essential oil. Microwave for around 30 to 60 seconds until the coconut oil is fully melted.

3. Pour the melted ingredients onto the dry or base ones. Then, use a mixing spoon or a whisk to stir your ingredients well. Make sure to mix as you slowly pour. You may even want to use your hand to ensure that the coconut oil fully amalgamates into the rest of the ingredients. Squeeze a handful of the texture and stick it together. It should feel like wet sand.

4. Pack your mixture firmly into the bath bomb mold. Open it and remove your bath bomb. If it starts to crack or fall apart, repack it into the mold.

5. Once you take it out, allow your bath bomb to dry for 24 hours. Then, seal it in an airtight bag or container.

Vibrant Bath Bomb ★★★☆☆

This cheerful bath bomb will definitely renew your child's love for baths. This recipe explains how you can make a bath bomb of three colors. Although, if you and your kid are up for a challenge, you can make a bath bomb that includes every color of the rainbow.

Ingredients

- Baking powder- 1 cup or 128g

- Fine sea salt- 1/2 cup or 64g

- Citric acid- 1/2 cup or 64g

- Corn starch- 1/2 cup or 64g

- Melted coconut oil- 2 1/2 tbsp

- Water- 2 tbsps

- Food coloring- 4 to 8 drops (make sure you have 3 food colorings of your choice).

Where to Find the Ingredients

You will find these ingredients at any local supermarket or convenience shop.

Directions

1. In a medium-sized bowl, place the citric acid, baking powder, and cornstarch. Mix all the ingredients well.

2. Mix the water and the coconut oil well together before slowly pouring them into the dry ingredients. Make sure to whisk consistently while you're adding the wet ingredients.

3. Make sure it feels like wet sand. If it's dry, add very little amounts of water.

4. Divide and separate the mixture into three bowls.

5. Add a few drops of each food coloring into each bowl and mix very well.

6. Generously fill up one side of the mold using the mixture in one of the bowls. Fill up the opposing side with another color mixture, and top it off, literally, with the third color.

7. Press the mold shut and allow it to sit for a few minutes. After you remove it, allow the bath bomb to dry well overnight.

Tips and Tricks:

- The humidity of the general environment may affect the consistency of your mixture. If this happens, add liquid as above. Make sure to use a pestle or spoon to get rid of any clumps that may appear in your "dough."

Substitutes:

- You can switch the fine sea salt with Epsom salt.
- You can add essential oils of your choice.

Surprise Toy Bath Bomb ★★★★☆

This recipe explains how you can make a bath bomb that includes a surprise toy for your child.

Ingredients

- Baking powder- 1 cup or 128g

- Epsom salts- 1/2 cup or 64g

- Citric acid- 1/2 cup or 64g

- Corn starch- 1/2 cup or 64g

- Ylang-Ylang- 2 tsp

- Your choice of food coloring- 4 to 8 drops (the number of drops depends on the shade you're aiming for).

- Magic grow animal pill

Where to Find the Ingredients

Find a trusted aromatherapy retailer to purchase these ingredients from. You will find the other ingredients at local convenience stores. You can also get the magic grow animal pill from any toy store.

Directions

1. Add all your dry ingredients into a large bowl and whisk to mix well.

2. In another bowl, pour your wet ingredients and mix properly.

3. Drop your liquid ingredients into the other bowl. Make sure to mix rapidly as you do so to prevent them from reacting.

4. Make sure your mixture feels like damp sand. Add your food coloring and mix well.

5. Pack half the bath bombs mold using the mixture. Place your animal grow pill in the middle and continue to fill the other half with the mixture.

6. Leave the mixture inside for a few minutes. Take it out and refrigerate your bath bomb for 24 hours.

7. Seal it in an airtight container until it's time to use it.

Tips and Tricks:
- You need to be quick to avoid any chemical reactions.

Substitutes:
- You can use Roman chamomile essential oil instead of Ylang-Ylang essential oil.

Citric Acid- Free Bath Bomb ★★★★★

Although this recipe is not overly challenging, it might get tricky since you're not using citric acid. Citric acid is a safe ingredient. However, if your child's skin is extra sensitive or you're worried about including acids in the recipe, you may feel more comfortable doing this DIY bath bomb.

Ingredients

- Baking powder- 2 cups or 256g

- Sweet almond oil- ⅛ cup 0r 16g

- Apple cider vinegar- 3 tbsp

- Your choice of essential oils- 1 tsp

- Your choice of food coloring- 4 to 8 drops (the number of drops depends on the shade you're aiming for).

- Dried flower petals- ¼ cup or 32g(optional)

- Sprinkles- ½ cup (optional)

Where to Find the Ingredients

Find these ingredients at any supermarket or convenience store. The essential oils can be bought from an aroma therapist, and the dried flower petals can be found on Amazon, Etsy, or at a florist.

Directions

1. In a large mixing bowl, sift the baking powder to remove all the lumps.

2. Add the sweet almond oil to the bowl and mix well.

3. In a separate bowl, mix your essential oils with the colorants. Add them to the baking powder.

4. Add the vinegar. Make sure to do it one step at a time and mix quickly to avoid it from reacting with the baking powder.

5. Press the mixture in your hands to make sure it feels like wet sand.

6. If you're using sprinkles and dried flower petals, add them in now.

7. Pack the mixture into the mold and hold it for a few minutes.

8. Take it out and leave it to dry for 24 hours.

Tips and Tricks:
- You need to be quick to avoid any chemical reactions.
- You can use warm bath water to amplify the fizzing effect.

Substitutes:
- You don't need to use the additives (sprinkles and dried flower petals).

Chapter 6: Bath Bombs that Soothe and Relax

Relaxation can be thought of as the best way of refreshing the mind and body. It's getting rid of tension and finding your way back to peace and equilibrium. Our bodies become revitalized when we are relaxing. When we relax, we give ourselves the chance to repair both mentally and physically.

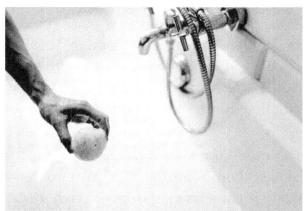

Your shoulder and neck area tend to tense up, you can get dizzy, get headaches, struggle with constant fatigue, and your sleep may be disrupted, all as a result of being overly stressed. Stress can also take a great toll on your mental well-being since it causes higher levels of cortisol, the stress hormone, to be produced in your body. Higher cortisol levels can affect your ability to focus and concentrate, make it more challenging to make decisions, cause you to worry, and have difficulty controlling your thoughts. Not being able to relax can make us feel irritable, stressed, anxious, possibly depressed, and may lower our self-esteem. We often involuntarily get highly defensive or aggressive, along with not communicating, avoiding certain situations, and this anxiety may trigger excess smoking and alcohol consumption. Allowing yourself to remain stressed for long periods can set off and worsen mood disorders.

While we can't always avoid stressful situations in our fast-paced lives, learning stress management and relaxation techniques is becoming more and more necessary. While stress can weigh you down, making you feel constantly fatigued, relaxation can improve blood flow, loosen tight muscles, and calm an overactive brain. There are techniques and tips which will help you get calmer and help clear your judgment. Besides being a conduit to aiding decision-making, and memory, relaxation can help you change your outlook on life and think more positively. You may also be surprised to learn that when you're relaxed, your body digests food more efficiently, which helps you absorb vital nutrients. This can help boost your immune system and improve your ability to fight off infection and disease. Avoiding stress and staying relaxed can help lower the risk of developing various mental and physical health problems.

When the word "relaxation" comes up, most people are quick to respond with, "I don't have the time." We erroneously believe that relaxation is not a priority. However, even when we don't have the time, we need to take the time to relax. In fact, if you underestimate the importance of resting or deprive your body of it, your body will inevitably take the long-overdue rest for you.

What many people don't realize is that they can incorporate rest into their daily routine quite easily by changing habits. While it's not always easy, staying consistent will allow you to make relaxation a habit and eventually turn it into a lifestyle. People relax in many different ways. What works for someone else may not necessarily work for you. Many people find that starting their day a little earlier helps them avoid setting off their morning on a rocky start. It also allows them to enjoy a hot cup of coffee or tea in the morning before they set off to work. Other people prefer to designate a specific time out of their day for relaxation.

To us, the best form of relaxation is indulging in self-care. That may be taking the time to prepare a soothing face mask each morning before you go about your day or taking just a few minutes to meditate before you go to bed. Better yet, you can prepare a relaxing bath with a softly-scented bath bomb, candles, and music twice a week. There is no better way to help you unwind and de-stress.

In this chapter, you will learn how making your own bath bombs can be the perfect way to de-stress and relax. You will find bath bomb recipes created especially for those who want to de-stress, soothe, relax, and calm their minds, bodies, and spirits.

Bath Bombs and Relaxation

Bath bombs can help you to doze off into a tranquil, peaceful sleep. When you take a few minutes to soak in warm water that's infused with relaxing and sleep-inducing essential oils like lavender, you are helping your body and calm down, which readies you for sleep. If you use the time you spend in the bath to free your mind, you'll free yourself of anxious and worrying thoughts, which keep you up at night. Using our phones or watching TV right before you go to sleep can stimulate your brain, making it harder to doze off. Additionally, when you step out of a cold bath and get exposed to colder air, this promotes the release of melatonin in the brain. Melatonin is a sleep-related hormone that can help you to fall asleep. In fact, many people may need to take melatonin pills in order to adjust to new time zones when they travel. Taking a warm bath with a bath bomb before you go to bed, however, can help your body produce melatonin in a natural way.

The common ingredients used in bath bombs, such as sea or Epsom salts, coconut oil, shea butter, and sunflower oil, will help deeply cleanse and moisturize your skin. You'll be left feeling very soft, pampered, and soothed after a really long day. Soaking in a warm bath can also stimulate blood flow to the surface of your skin. This, combined with the ingredients we discussed, can make your skin look refreshed and more youthful. The bath will also encourage your arteries and veins to expand temporarily, which would lower your blood pressure. All these benefits are so easily achieved to de-stress, regain your composure, and maintain peace.

Each essential oil targets a certain issue or is used for a specific purpose. For instance, Roman chamomile essential oil works to calm the mind. Rose essential oil can help reduce anxiety and promote a younger complexion, and myrrh can help with acne and other skin problems. The recipes in this chapter include ingredients and essential oils that will help you relax. The overall scent of the bath bomb can also influence your state of mind, energy levels, and level of relaxation.

Finally, bath bombs give a lush, luxurious, and opulent feel. You can forget about all your worries just by dropping one into the bath and watching it dissolve into the water. Bath bombs can turn any ordinary task into a relaxing and joyful experience. The following are some bath bomb recipes tailored to help put your mind and body at ease:

Soothe and Relax Bath Bomb

This basic yet highly relaxing bath bomb recipe will leave you soothed and relaxed. It will take no more than five minutes to prepare, leaving you with around five large bath bombs to enjoy whenever you need to unwind.

Ingredients

- Baking powder- 1 cup or 128g
- Citric acid- ½ cup or 64g
- Cornstarch- ½ cup or 64g
- Epsom salts- ½ cup or 64g
- Water- ¾ tsp
- Essential oil of your choice- 2 tsp
- Oil of your choice- 2 tsp
- Food coloring of your choice- 5 drops (you can add more depending on the intensity of the shade you want)
- Additions of your choice (dried flower petals, sugar cake decorations, etc....)

Where to Find the Ingredients

You can find these ingredients at your local aroma therapist or convenience store.

Directions

1. Mix all your dry ingredients into a large bowl, except for the citric acid.

2. Grab a jar with a lid and pour all your liquid ingredients inside. Seal tightly and shake well to mix all your ingredients together.

3. Then, pour your liquid ingredients into the large bowl with the dry ingredients. Use your hand to mix all your ingredients together. Once done, add your citric

acid. Your mixture will start fizzing, which is a normal reaction due to the citric acid. You don't have to panic.

4. Hold the mixture into your hand and press lightly to make sure it holds its shape. It should feel like wet sand.

5. Place your mixture into your mold and press down firmly. You may want to overfill your mold a little to ensure that it holds together well. Hold your mixture into the mold for a few minutes before taking it out.

6. Take the bath bomb out of the mold and leave it to harden and dry overnight on a tray covered with wax paper.

7. To be sure, give them a day or two to let them set before you use them.

Tips and Tricks:

- Don't use too much water as the bath bomb will lose its fizz that way, especially after you add your citric acid.
- Press your mixture down really tightly using a spoon or spatula to make sure that it holds.

Substitutes:

- Use eucalyptus, rose, lavender, lemongrass, or orange essential oils for the best results. You can use more than one; however, make sure that the amounts don't mess with the overall consistency.
- Use jojoba, olive, baby oil, coconut, or sweet almond oil for the best results.

It's Bedtime Bath Bomb

If you haven't had a good night's sleep in a long time, this bath bomb is the perfect way to remedy the situation. This recipe only takes 10 minutes to prepare and leaves you with six large bath bombs to enjoy. Not only will it make you drift off to sleep in no time, but it will also leave you smelling delicious.

Ingredients

- Baking powder- 1 cup 128g
- Citric acid- ½ cup or 64g
- Cornstarch- ¾ cup or 96g
- Epsom salts- ½ cup or 64g
- Almond oil- 2 tbsp
- Witch hazel- 3 tsp
- Lavender mica powder- ½ tsp
- Breathe or any other respiratory essential oil-5 drops
- Chamomile essential oil- 8 drops
- Lavender essential oil- 8 drops
- Magnesium powder- 1 tsp
- Spray bottle with water

Where to Find the Ingredients

Visit your local organic shop, convenience store, or aromatherapists to shop for the ingredients.

Directions

1. Combine all the dry ingredients in a large bowl and mix them very well. Make sure you are left with no clumps.

2. Pour your essential oils, almond oil, and witch hazel into a separate small glass bowl. Make sure that you whisk them very well.

3. Pour your wet ingredients into the large bowl. Your mixture should start fizzing up once your liquid touches the dry ingredients.

4. Use your hands or a fork to mix everything. Your mixture should feel like damp sand.

5. Bring your bath bomb molds and start filling them up halfway. Make sure you press the mixture down hard into the mold. You can use a spatula for this.

6. Then, use the spray bottle to spray a bit of water. One spray will do and then press down once again to ensure they're firm.

7. Seal the mold carefully and press it down firmly.

8. Let it sit on your counter for 24 hours to dry before you take it out.

Tips and Tricks:
- Don't use too much water, as the bath bomb will lose its fizz that way.
- You need to press your mixture down really well to make sure that it holds.

Substitutes:
- Use the mica powder of your choice. Though, lavender is known to have calming effects and a luxurious feel.

Sit Back and Meditate ★★☆☆☆

If you like to meditate or do yoga, this bath bomb is the perfect way to begin or finish off your meditation session. Even if you don't plan on actively meditating, the "sit back and meditate bath bomb" will allow you to gently bring serenity and peace to your mind. This fragrant creation will help you visualize, bring attention to your sensations, and align yourself with your thoughts and feelings. This recipe will only take a few minutes to put together and will make around five large bath bombs.

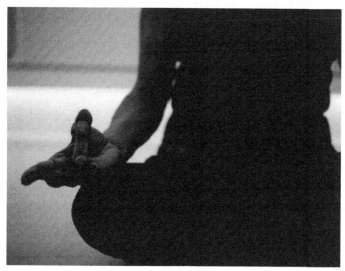

Ingredients

- Baking powder- 1 cup or 128g
- Citric acid- ½ cup or 64g
- Epsom salts- 3 tbsp
- Cornstarch- ½ cup or 64g
- Unrefined coconut oil- 3 tsp
- Mica powder (optional)- ½ tsp
- Cedarwood essential oil- 5 drops
- Frankincense essential oil- 5 drops

- Lavender essential oil- 4 drops

- Ylang-ylang essential oil- 2 drops

- Sweet orange essential oil- 4 drops

Where to Find the Ingredients

You can get your ingredients at a convenience store and an aromatherapist.

Directions

1. In a large bowl, combine the citric acid, corn starch, Epsom salts, and baking soda. If you want your bath bomb to have a certain color, add your choice of mica powder at this stage and combine everything thoroughly.

2. Melt the coconut oil in the microwave and pour it into your dry mixture.

3. Then, pour your essential oils into a bowl and mix very well. Make sure you break down the clumps with your fingers or a spoon. You can also sift it.

4. You can keep a reserve of essential oils in a spray bottle if needed. Spray it into the mixture until you reach your desired consistency. It should feel like wet sand.

5. Hold the mixture in your hand. Press on it lightly and make sure it's doesn't fall apart and crumble.

6. Place and press the mixture firmly into your molds.

7. Leave your bath bomb in the mold overnight to harden and dry. If you have a metal mold, carefully take it out before you leave it to dry.

Tips and Tricks:
- Don't spray more than two sprays at a time.
- If you spray too much, it will start to fizz. You don't want to wet your mixture; you want to dampen it.

Substitutes:
- Keep to the recipe for this one, as the combination of essential oils is particularly fragrant and relaxing.

Stress-Relief Bath Bomb

This bath bomb combines ingredients that can help immediately lift your mood and reduce your stress and anxiety. In only 15 minutes, you can easily make an incredible bath bomb that chases all your worries away. The best thing about this recipe is that it makes four huge bath bombs!

Ingredients

- Baking powder- 1 cup or 128g
- Citric acid- ½ cup or 64g
- Cornstarch- ¾ cup or 96g
- Epsom salts- ½ cup of 64g
- Almond oil- 2 tbsp
- Witch hazel- 3 tsp
- Green or blue mica powder- ½ tsp
- Grapefruit essential oil- 10 drops
- Citrus essential oil- 10 drops
- Clary sage essential oil- 6 to 8 drops
- Chamomile essential oil- 8 to 10 drops
- Lavender essential oil- 8 to 10 drops
- Spray bottle with water

Where to Find the Ingredients

Search a nearby convenience store and aromatherapists for the ingredients.

Directions

1. Gather all your dry ingredients in a large bowl and mix them very well. Make sure you are left with no clumps.

2. Pour the essential oils, almond oil, and witch hazel into a separate small bowl and whisk them well.

3. Combine your wet ingredients into the large bowl. Don't panic! Your mixture will start fizzing.

4. Use your hands or a fork to mix everything. You should be left with a moist, sandy mixture.

5. Bring your bath bomb molds and start filling them up halfway with a spatula. Press your formula down to hold it in place. Then, use the spray bottle to spray a bit of water (just once) and press down once again to ensure they're firm.

6. Seal the mold carefully and press it down firmly.

7. Let it sit on your counter for 24 hours to dry before you take it out.

Tips and Tricks:
- Too much water can make the bath bomb lose its frizz. One spray is enough.
- If you don't press the bath bomb into the mold well, it will not hold together.

Substitutes:
- You can switch the citrus essential oil with orange essential oil.
- Use the mica powder of your choice. However, blue and green have the most relaxing and calming effects.

Let Go and Unwind Bath Bomb

This bath bomb helps create the perfect environment in which you can unwind. Watching the bath bomb dissolve into the water and inhaling its aromatic scent is enough to help you let go of all unwanted thoughts and worries. This recipe is very easy to make. With a prep time of just 10 minutes, you can make seven bath bombs to enjoy whenever your heart desires.

Ingredients

- Baking powder- 4 cups or 512g
- Citric acid- 2 cups or 256g
- Epsom salts- ½ cup or 64g
- Borage oil- ¼ cup or 32g
- Polysorbate 80- 4 tsp
- Lilac liquid soap dye- ½ tsp
- Lavender essential oil- 8 to 10 drops
- Spray bottle with witch hazel
- Dried lavender

Where to Find the Ingredients

You can get your ingredients at a convenience store and an aromatherapist. Polysorbate 80 is available on Amazon.

Directions

1. Pour your borage oil, polysorbate 80, lavender essential oil, and lilac liquid soap dye into a small container and mix very well using a spoon. Keep in mind that your colorant may not fully amalgamate with the rest of your mixture, which is fine.

2. Grab a large container to place your citric acid and baking soda. Mix well, and then sift the mixture to get rid of any clumps or break them up using your fingers. Stir the ingredients gently once again.

3. Add your wet ingredients to the large container and mix thoroughly with your hands.

4. The consistency of your mixture should be similar to that of wet sand. It should also maintain its shape if you squeeze it. It will crumble if it's too dry. In that case, you need to spray witch hazel into the mix. Keep spraying until you reach the desired consistency.

5. Place a pinch of dried lavender into the center of the mold and then fill up both halves using your mixture. Press down, so it firms up.

6. Press both halves of the mold to each other to hold them together.

7. While twisting, gently pull up the top half of the mold. Do the same to the other end.

8. Put your bath bomb on the counter and allow it to harden and dry overnight.

Tips and Tricks:
- Don't spray more witch hazel than you need.

Substitutes:
- You can add essential oils of your choice. Though, make sure not to mess up the entire consistency of your recipe.
- Use the mica powder of your choice.

There are endless benefits to relaxation. Indulging in self-care from time to time is crucial to the maintenance of your mental and physical health. Making your own bath bomb and using it is the perfect way to combat stress and promote mental and physical relaxation.

Chapter 7: Bath Bombs for Each Skin Type

When buying cosmetics or skin care products, an important consideration is whether a product or its ingredients will suit your skin type or not. If you use products designed for a skin type different from yours, you'll not only be disappointed with the results but will also possibly have to deal with nasty skin reactions. The same goes for when you're creating homemade skin products, in this case, bath bombs. Even the slightest error when creating them or using ingredients you haven't tried before could lead to severe allergies and undesirable skin reactions.

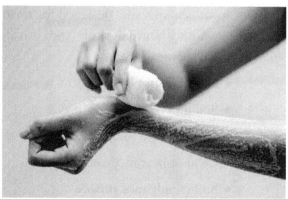

Imagine the horror of finding your skin has dried out after a self-care session – and not knowing why! That is why it's imperative to know your skin type before you buy, or more importantly, when you make skin care products at home. Bath bombs are no exception. While they are used mainly to make your baths more luxurious, they can have other wonderful properties. In addition to bringing colors and pleasant fragrances to your bath, bath bombs can also leave your skin with a fresh glow by moisturizing and nourishing it.

However, if you use a bath bomb that doesn't suit you, it could lead to problems ranging from dryness, skin irritation, and itchiness to severe allergic reactions. This chapter will give an insight into how you can identify your skin type and the different bath bomb formulations you can try that are designed specifically for different skin types. So, whether you have sensitive, dry, or oily skin, keep on reading to find a bath bomb recipe that works best for you and your skin.

Normal Skin

Normal skin has very few issues and is the most common skin type people have. If you're someone whose skin type is normal, then you're luckily considered to have good skin that doesn't require extra care, unlike the other skin types. Nonetheless, it's still prudent to use products specially designed for normal skin to avoid any nasty reactions. Normal skin type usually has the following tell-tale characteristics.

- Soft and supple to the touch
- Small pores on the skin
- Not sensitive to the usual environment
- Clear appearance and coloring
- Sufficiently moisturized

For normal skin, you want to create a bath bomb that doesn't leave your skin too dry or too oily. You don't want to be dealing with skin problems after a luxurious bath. Here are two recipes for bath bombs you can try making at home that are perfect for normal skin.

Milk and Honey DIY Bath Bombs

This milk and honey combination bath bomb can be a great addition to your bath time routine. It not only hydrates and nourishes but also helps exfoliate your skin, and the result is fresh, luminous-looking skin. The addition of cocoa butter to the recipe ensures that your skin gets hydrated, whereas milk and honey have numerous undeniable skin benefits.

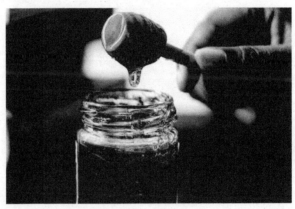

Ingredients

- Baking soda - 2 cups or 256g
- Citric acid - 1 ¼ cups or 160g
- Cornstarch - ½ cup or 64g
- Cocoa butter - 65g
- Goat milk powder - 65g
- Honey powder - 25g
- Mica powder - 1 to 2 tsp
- Polysorbate 80 - 1 tsp
- Essential oil blend - 10g

Where to Find Ingredients

You can easily find the main ingredients at any market near you. If you can't find cocoa butter, you can substitute it with shea butter used in the same quantity. The milk powder can also be changed according to your preference. For the essential oil blend, you can try a combination of vanilla oleoresin and cardamom, or lavender and chamomile.

Directions

1.Let the cocoa butter melt in a double boiler or microwave for one-minute intervals until melted.

2.Let the melted butter cool off for around ten minutes before adding the essential oil blend and polysorbate.

3.Next, mix the citric acid with baking soda in a separate bowl.

4.Add honey powder, milk powder, and mica to the mix. Stir it well to combine the ingredients properly.

5.Now, mix the two bowls containing the wet and dry ingredients together until you achieve a damp sand-like mixture.

6.Fill this mixture into bath bomb molds, and create a high dome shape in the middle. Press the mold halves together tightly and wipe away any excess material.

7.Unmold the bath bomb carefully and place it on a baking tray lined with bubble wrap and allow it to dry for about a day.

Tips and Tricks

1. Make sure you add the liquid ingredients one teaspoon at a time to avoid any sort of reaction when making the bath bomb.
2. The quantity of cocoa butter used depends on the humidity in your area. Extreme humidity can make it difficult to shape the bath bombs, so make sure to rehydrate the mixture with alcohol or witch hazel if you see it drying out when you put it into the mold.

Ingredient Substitutions

Cocoa butter	Shea butter
Goat milk powder	Coconut milk powder
Essential Oils – lavender/ chamomile	Vanilla oleoresin/ cardamom

Fresh Orange DIY Bath Bombs

This bath bomb is best for a fresh, nice bath on a hot summer day. It will leave you feeling calm and relaxed after your bath. In addition, it also helps relieve sore muscles and, of course, moisturizes your skin.

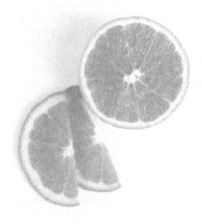

Ingredients

- Baking soda – 1 cup or 128g
- Citric acid – ½ cup or 64g
- Epsom salts – ½ cup or 64g
- Cornstarch – ½ cup or 64g
- Mica powder – 1 to 2 tsp
- Dried orange peel – 1 tsp
- Essential oil blend – 10g
- Coconut oil – 5g
- Water – as needed

Where to Find Ingredients

Most of these ingredients can be found in your kitchen. If not, cornstarch and baking soda can be found in the baking section of your grocery store. Epsom salts can be found online or in the pharmacy section of a grocery store. To make dried orange peel, zest three oranges and allow the zest to dry for two days, or you can also find this in the spice section of a grocery store. For the essential oil blend, you can use any fragrance you like. Orange essential oil mixed with tea tree and lavender essential oils works best for this recipe.

Directions

1. Combine the dry ingredients in a bowl first; these include baking soda, citric acid, Epsom salt, corn starch, and mica powder.

2. Whisk all the ingredients together, so they are well mixed together.

3. In another bowl, add melted coconut oil, water, and your essential oil blend and whisk.

4. Slowly pour the liquid mixture into the dry one, being careful that the mixture does not fizz too much.

5. Add the dried orange peels to the mix.

6. Stir and combine the mixture until it looks like damp sand.

7. Press the mixture into the two halves of the bath bomb mold you're using. Close the container tightly and remove any excess air.

8. Allow this mixture to dry for 24 hours, then remove the mold.

Tips and Tricks

1. Make sure you add the liquid ingredients one teaspoon at a time to avoid any sort of reaction when making the bath bomb.
2. You can tweak the essential oil combinations and the mica powder you use to change the fragrances and colors of the bath bomb.

Ingredient Substitutions

Epsom salts	Any other sea salt
Essential Oils – lavender/ tea tree oil	Vanilla/ fruity essential oils

Dry Skin

Dry skin could be caused by a genetic disorder or simply haphazard skincare habits. But for most people, there's no apparent reason for it. Dry skin gives rise to many skin issues and requires extra care and attention. As dry skin can be extra sensitive to environmental factors, it's essential that you choose only products and ingredients that suit your skin. The following characteristics are attributed to dry skin.

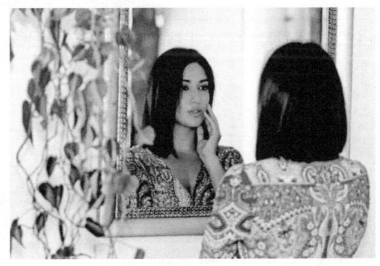

- Skin feels tight
- Irritation and itchiness
- Fine lines and small pores are visible
- Flaky, white skin
- Makeup doesn't adhere properly

For dry skin, you want to create a bath bomb that doesn't make your skin dry out or get irritated. Winters, especially, are worse for those with dry skin. A hot bath seems nice until you've to deal with the aftermath of the bath in the form of extreme dryness. These two recipes for bath bombs are proven to nourish and moisturize dry skin and leave your skin feeling supple and soft after a bath.

Soothing Oatmeal and Lavender DIY Bath Bombs

Oatmeal has been used for centuries as a skin care product to moisturize dry skin, reduce inflammation and irritation. This bath bomb is the perfect way to relax, enjoy and ease your skin troubles all in one. It will, without a doubt, soothe dry skin, relax your muscles, and suck away all your stress on any given day.

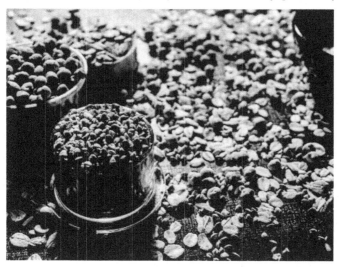

Ingredients

- Baking soda – ½ cup or 64g
- Colloidal oatmeal – ⅛ cup or 16g
- Citric acid – ¼ cup or 32g
- Epsom salts – ⅛ cup or 16g
- Sweet almond oil – 3 tsp
- Rolled oats – 2 tbsp
- Chamomile essential oil – 10 drops
- Witch hazel – 1 to 2 tsp

Where to Find the Ingredients

You can easily find the main ingredients at any market near you. If not, cornstarch and baking soda can be found in the baking section of your grocery store. Epsom salts can be found online or in the pharmacy section of a grocery store. Rolled oats can also be found online or in a grocery store. If you can't find witch hazel, you can use water as an alternative.

Directions

1. Combine the dry ingredients together in a bowl – these will include baking soda, colloidal oatmeal, citric acid, and Epsom salts.

2. Whisk these ingredients together properly to ensure no clumps are left in the mixture.

3. Next, combine the wet ingredients in a separate bowl by mixing the essential oils together with water or witch hazel.

4. Now, slowly pour the wet ingredients into the dry ones and stir as you go. If the mixture suddenly starts to foam, slow down.

5. After whisking completely, scoop a small amount of the mixture into your hands to test its consistency and adherence. If the mixture sticks well, then proceed; otherwise, hydrate it by adding a few drops of water or witch hazel.

6. Before putting the mixture into the molds, place one pinch of rolled oats at the base of the mold.

7. Press the mixture into both halves and close the mold tightly. Remove any excess.

8. Once the mixture is set, remove the bath bomb from the mold and let it dry for eight hours, then store it in a cool, dry place.

Tips and Tricks
1. Make sure you add the liquid ingredients one teaspoon at a time to avoid any sort of reaction when making the bath bomb. 2. If you add both solutions at once, the powders will fizz out of the bowl and be wasted.

Ingredient Substitutions	
Epsom salts	Any other sea salt
Essential Oils – chamomile	Lavender

Ultra-Hydrating Coconut DIY Bath Bombs

This bath bomb recipe is a real treat for you and your loved ones' skin, as coconut oil is said to be the best treatment for dry and dull skin. The best part about these bath bombs is that they can be made with only eight ingredients and are completely non-toxic and organic, meaning they are safe to use by all your family members, even your little ones.

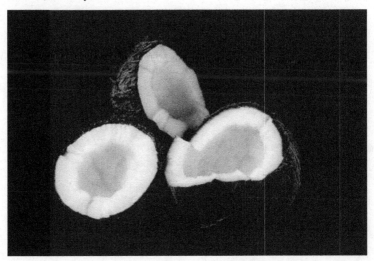

Ingredients

- Baking soda – ½ cup or 64g
- Citric acid – ¼ cup or 32 g
- Epsom salts – ¼ cup or 160
- Cornstarch – ¼ cup or 32g
- Mica powder – ¼ tsp
- Fractionated coconut oil – 1 tbsp
- Essential oil blend – 20 drops
- Coconut oil – 5g
- Water – 1 tbsp

Where to Find the Ingredients

Most of these ingredients can be easily found in your kitchen. If not, cornstarch and baking soda can be found in the baking section of your grocery store. Epsom salts can be found online or in the pharmacy section of a grocery store.

Directions

1. Combine the dry ingredients in a bowl first; these include baking soda, citric acid, Epsom salts, cornstarch, and mica powder.

2. Whisk all the dry ingredients together to get a uniform mixture.

3. In another bowl, add melted coconut oil, water, and essential oil blend and whisk it into a uniform mixture.

4. Slowly pour the liquid mixture into the dry one slowly, so the mixture does not fizz too much.

5. Stir and mix the combination until it looks like damp sand.

6. Press the mixture into the two halves of the bath bomb mold you're using. Close the container tightly and remove any excess.

7. Allow this mixture to dry for six hours, then remove the mold and let the bath bombs dry.

8. Dry for eight hours, then store in a cool, dry place.

Tips and Tricks

1. Make sure you add the liquid ingredients one teaspoon at a time to avoid any sort of reaction when making the bath bomb.
2. Ensure that you store these bath bombs in an airtight container or jar so that they're not exposed to moisture.

Ingredient Substitutions

Epsom salts	Any other sea salt
Essential Oils – Coconut oil	Almond oil

Oily Skin

Oily skin is pretty common these days because of environmental factors which cause an accumulation of dirt, dust, and oil in our skin. Although some moisture is necessary for our skin (otherwise, our skin gets dry and cracked), too much can be just as bad as too little. The main characteristics of oily skin are:

- Shiny and oily appearance
- Pores are enlarged
- Wrinkles and lines are less visible
- Makeup rubs off easily

For oily skin, you want to create a bath bomb that doesn't make your skin too moisturized and that leaves it oily. Acne and pimples often go along with oily skin and are a condition no one wants. It is therefore really important to select or make a bath bomb that complements and enhances your skin. So, here are two recipes for bath bombs you can try making at home that work perfectly for oily skin.

Mango Butter DIY Bath Bombs

This simple bath bomb recipe is perfect for oily skin; it contains butter and spinach powder – both of which are famous for their anti-aging effects on the skin. Moreover, the other ingredients ensure that the natural essential oils in your skin are not depleted after a bath and so help prevent oily skin and acne.

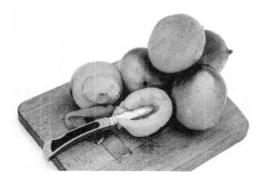

Ingredients

- Baking soda - 1 cup or 128g
- Citric acid - ½ cup or 64 g
- Cornstarch - ½ cup or 64 g
- Spinach powder - 1 tbsp
- Mango butter - 4 tbsp
- Arrowroot powder - ½ tbsp
- French green clay - ½ tbsp
- Liquid carrier oil - as needed
- Lemon grass essential oil - 2 ml
- Palmarosa essential oil - 1 ml
- Witch hazel - As needed
- Bergamot essential oil - 1 ml

Where to Find the Ingredients

You can easily find the main ingredients at any market near you. If not, cornstarch and baking soda can be found in the baking section of your grocery store. Green clay and spinach powder can be found through any online retailer, while essential oils are readily available both online and in markets.

Directions

1. Weigh the mango butter on a scale before putting it in a microwavable container. Heat at 30% power in the microwave or double boiler until completely melted.

2. Add the essential oil blend into the mango butter and stir until completely mixed together.

3. In a separate container, add the dry ingredients that include citric acid, baking soda, spinach powder, French green clay, and arrowroot powder and mix them thoroughly.

4. Now add the wet and dry ingredients together slowly. Whisk the mixture until completely merged together, and it feels like damp sand.

5. Fill this mixture into bath bomb molds, creating the middle hump. Press the mold halves together tightly and wipe away any extra material.

6. Unmold the bath bomb carefully, and place it on a baking tray lined with bubble wrap. Allow it to dry for about a day.

Tips and Tricks
1. Make sure you add the liquid ingredients one teaspoon at a time to avoid any sort of reaction when making the bath bomb.
2. Ensure that you store these bath bombs in an airtight container or jar so that they're not exposed to moisture.

Ingredient Substitutions	
Epsom salts	Any other sea salt
Essential Oils – Coconut oil	Almond oil

Therapeutic Clay DIY Bath Bombs

Clay bath bombs are perfect for a therapeutic skin care experience that leaves your skin feeling fresh and nourished. Clays are used in skin care for their impressive purifying and healing qualities. These clay bath bombs deep clean the pores on your skin by pulling the oil from them and leaving your skin feeling refreshed, clean, and nourished.

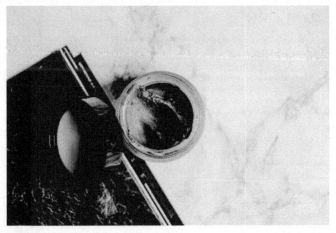

Ingredients

- Baking soda – 1 cup or 128g
- Citric acid – 1 cup or 128g
- Cornstarch – ½ cup or 64g
- Epsom salts – 1 cup or 128g
- Clay minerals – 1 cup or 128g
- French green clay – ½ tbsp
- Liquid carrier oil – as needed
- Essential oil blend – 15 drops
- Witch hazel – As needed
- Mica powder – optional

Where to Find the Ingredients

Most of these ingredients can be easily found in your kitchen. If not, cornstarch and baking soda can be found in the baking section of your grocery store. Epsom salts can be found online or in the pharmacy section of a grocery store. Carrier and essential oils can be chosen based on your preferences.

Directions

1. Combine the dry ingredients in a bowl first – these include baking soda, citric acid, Epsom salts, cornstarch, and mica powder.

2. Whisk all the ingredients together to get a uniform mixture.

3. In another bowl, add the wet ingredients together and whisk them into a uniform mixture.

4. Slowly pour the liquid mixture into the dry one so that the mixture does not fizz too much.

5. Add the clay minerals to the mix.

6. Stir and mix the combination until it looks like damp sand.

7. Press the mixture into the two halves of the bath bomb mold you're using. Close the container tightly and remove any excess.

8. Allow this mixture to dry for a day, then remove the mold.

Tips and Tricks
1. To avoid any form of reaction when making the bath bomb, add the liquid ingredients one teaspoon at a time. 2. To modify the aromas and colors of the bath bomb, you can experiment with different essential oil mixtures and mica powder.

Ingredient Substitutions	
French Green Clay	Bentonite Clay
Witch Hazel	Water

Chapter 8: Fruity and Floral Bath Bombs

Bath bombs aren't just for kids; in fact, they're hugely popular among both women and men who prefer a luxuriously-relaxing bath instead of a simple shower. One of the best things about these products is their versatility – the numerous scents and colors they're available in. Not to generalize, but women specifically love floral and fruity scents, whether it's for their perfumes, lotions, shampoos, or body wash. Bath bombs are no exception to this. Although there's a huge range of bath bombs available in the market, the satisfaction that comes from making your own floral and fruity scented bath bombs outweighs anything else. Not to mention the money you save. A big plus is that when you use homemade bath bombs, there's less chance of skin allergies, and you can modify the scents and flavors according to your preferences and skin type.

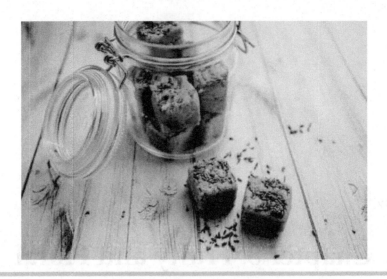

Fruity Bath Bombs

Fruity bath bombs provide a fresh, fruity scent and are also nutritious for your skin. The best part about making your own fruity bath bombs is that you can use completely organic fruits instead of the artificial scents added to commercial bath bombs. Listed below are some of the best fruity bath bombs you can make at home.

Strawberry

This strawberry bath bomb recipe is one of the best-smelling and nutritious recipes because it uses real strawberries. By using real strawberries, the bath bombs will be authentically colored and scented. Strawberries are said to be very good for your skin, but using solid pieces of strawberry would be difficult to clean up. This recipe solves that problem and uses dehydrated strawberries in powder form. Another important ingredient for this recipe is the strawberry perfume oil that gives a sweet smell to the mixture.

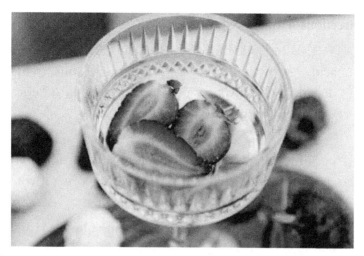

Ingredients

- Baking soda - 2 cups or 256g
- Citric acid - 1 cup or 128g
- Cornstarch - ⅓ cup or 45g
- Epsom salt - ⅓ cup or 45g
- Strawberry perfume oil - 1.5 tsp
- Almond oil - 2 tbsp
- Mica powder - 1 to 2 tsp
- Dehydrated strawberry powder - 2 tbsp
- Witch Hazel - As needed

Where to Find the Ingredients

Most of these ingredients can be easily found in your kitchen. Cornstarch and baking soda can be found in the baking section of your grocery store. Epsom salts can be found online or in the pharmacy store. To make strawberry powder, dehydrate strawberry slices by freeze-drying them, then crush them in a blender to form fine powder particles. It's important to crush the strawberry pieces into a very fine powder; otherwise, they'll swell up and be difficult to remove from your bathtub after your bath.

Directions

1. Whisk all the dry ingredients (baking soda, citric acid, cornstarch, Mica powder, Epsom salt, and dehydrated strawberry powder) together in a large bowl until completely mixed.

2. Pour the wet ingredients (Almond oil, strawberry perfume oil, witch hazel) in a small jar with a lid and shake it well to mix them. Add food coloring if you want the bath bomb to have a bright color.

3. Mix the two bowls containing the wet and dry ingredients together, adding the wet to the dry until you achieve a damp sand-like mixture. Use your hands to knead the mixture if you want to achieve a consistent mixture.

4. Fill this mixture into bath bomb molds, and make a high heap in the middle. Press the mold halves together tightly and wipe away any residue.

5. After ten to twenty minutes, unmold the bath bomb carefully and place it on a baking tray lined with bubble wrap and allow it to dry for a day or two.

Tips and Tricks

1. Make sure you add the liquid ingredients one teaspoon at a time to avoid any sort of reaction when making the bath bomb.
2. Slowly keep stirring with the whisk to activate the citric acid; if it starts to fizz too much, slow down.
3. Extreme humidity can make it difficult to shape the bath bombs, so make sure to rehydrate the mixture with alcohol or witch hazel if you see it drying out when you put it into the mold.

Ingredient Substitutions

Epsom Salts	Any other sea salt
Almond Oil	Any other nut oil
Witch Hazel	Water

Forest Berries

This fruity bath bomb contains a sweet mixture of dried forest berries and a perfect essential oil blend for a sweet, fresh scent. A great part about this bath bomb recipe is that you can modify the colors according to your own taste and use whatever berries you like the most. You can also use a mixture of them. This bath bomb recipe is said to be moisturizing, great for dry skin, and leaves your skin smelling like forest berries.

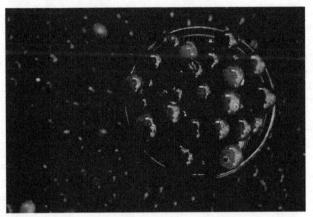

Ingredients

- Baking soda – 2 cups or 256g
- Citric acid – 1 ¼ cups or 160g
- Cornstarch – ½ cup or 64g
- Coconut oil – 65g
- Mica powder – 1 to 2 tsp
- Polysorbate 80 – 1 tsp
- Dead sea salt – 1 cup
- Essential oil blend – 10g
- Forest berries fruit tea – 4 bags

Where to Find the Ingredients

Some of these ingredients are not commonly found in your kitchen. However, you can easily find them on Amazon or through local vendors. The mica powder is your colorant. For the essential oil blend, you can try a combination of lavender and chamomile with perfume oil to get that berry scent.

Directions

1. First, mix all the dry ingredients (Baking soda, citric acid, Dead Sea salt, corn starch, mica powder) together in a large bowl.

2. Add the dehydrated and crushed berries into the mixture and whisk until combined completely.

3. Melt coconut oil in the microwave in a separate container.

4. In the separate container (#3, above), add the forest berry tea with an essential oil blend of your choice. Add polysorbate to the mix and stir.

5. Now, combine the contents of the two containers together slowly.

6. Knead the mixture together until you obtain a damp mixture.

7. Put this mixture into bath bomb molds, ensure to create a high heap in the middle. Press the mold halves together tightly and wipe away any extra material.

8. Unmold the bath bomb carefully, and place it on a baking tray lined with bubble wrap, allowing it to dry for about a day or two.

Tips and Tricks

1. Make sure you add the liquid ingredients one teaspoon at a time to avoid any sort of reaction when making the bath bomb.
2. Ensure the berry powder is crushed into fine particles.
3. The quantity of coconut oil depends on how humid your atmosphere is.
4. Extreme humidity can make it difficult to shape the bath bombs, so make sure to rehydrate the mixture with alcohol or witch hazel if you see it drying out when you put it into the mold.

Ingredient Substitutions

Coconut oil	Almond oil
Dead sea salt	Epsom salts

Fruity Mix

Similar to the forest berries recipe, this bath bomb recipe makes use of freeze-dried fruits to obtain the scent and color of the bath bomb. The many fruits used in this mixture add to the luxurious feeling of your skin after a bath. The fruits include lemon, orange, citrus, and berries. The best part about this recipe is the amazing scent because of the unique, essential oil blend used.

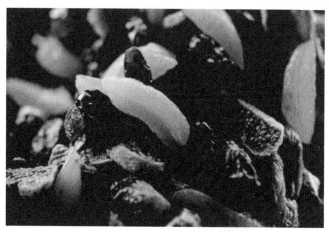

Ingredients

- Baking soda – 2 cups or 256g
- Citric acid – 1 cup or 128g
- Cornstarch – ½ cup or 64g
- Fractionated coconut oil – 1 cup or 128g
- Mica powder – 1 to 2 tsp
- Polysorbate 80 – 1 tsp
- Dried Fruit Mix Powder – ½ cup or 64g
- Essential oil blend – 15g

Where to Find the Ingredients

You can easily find the main ingredients at any market near you. Cornstarch and baking soda can be found in the baking section of your grocery store. Epsom salts can be found online or in the pharmacy store. To make the fruit mix powder, dehydrate fruit slices by freeze-drying them, then crush them in a blender to form fine powder particles. It's important to crush the fruit pieces into a very fine powder, or otherwise, they'll swell up and be difficult to remove from your bathtub later.

Directions

1. Mix all the dry ingredients (baking soda, citric acid, cornstarch, Mica powder, Epsom salts, and dehydrated fruit powder) together in a large bowl until completely mixed.

2. Pour the wet ingredients (Almond oil, essential oil blend, witch hazel) into a small jar and shake well to mix them.

3. Now, mix the two bowls containing the wet and dry ingredients together until you achieve a damp sand-like mixture.

4. Place this mixture into the two halves of the bath bomb molds, making sure to create a heap in the middle. Press the mold halves together tightly and wipe away any excess.

5. After ten minutes, unmold the bath bomb carefully and allow it to dry for 24 hours.

Tips and Tricks
1. Make sure you add the liquid ingredients one teaspoon at a time to avoid any sort of reaction when making the bath bomb.
2. The essential oil blend used for this recipe should be as follows:

<table>
<tr><td colspan="2">• Lime essential oil – 5 drops</td></tr>
<tr><td colspan="2">• Lemon essential oil – 4 drops</td></tr>
<tr><td colspan="2">• Orange essential oil – 4 drops</td></tr>
<tr><td colspan="2">• Tangerine essential oil – 3 drops</td></tr>
<tr><td colspan="2">• Spearmint essential oil – 2 drops</td></tr>
<tr><td colspan="2">Ingredient Substitutions</td></tr>
<tr><td>Fractionated coconut oil</td><td>Almond oil</td></tr>
</table>

Lemon Vanilla ★★★☆☆

This lemon vanilla bath bomb recipe is best for a fizzy, refreshing, and uplifting bath after a long day. It has both lemon and vanilla essential oils to make the refreshing, delicious scent, plus lemon peels for the major skin benefits it provides. The dried lemon peels not only nourish your skin but also give an aesthetic look to the bath bomb when it's finished.

Ingredients

- Baking soda - 1 cup or 128g
- Citric acid - ½ cup or 64g
- Cornstarch - ½ cup or 64g
- Epsom salts- 3 tbsp
- Coconut Oil - 2 tsp
- Lemon essential oil - 15 drops
- Vanilla essential oil - 10 drops
- Dried lemon zest - 2 to 3 tbsp
- Witch hazel - ¾ tsp

Where to Find the Ingredients

You can find baking soda and citric acid easily in a grocery store. If you have a hard time finding citric acid, you can likely find it online. Dried lemon zest can either be made at home or found in the spice section of your nearest grocery store. Essential oils can be bought from local vendors or online.

Directions

1. Combine the dry ingredients in a large container and whisk them together thoroughly. These should include cornstarch, baking powder, citric acid, lemon zest, and Epsom salts.

2. Next, blend the essential oils together and add them to melted coconut oil. To dilute the solution, add witch hazel in suitable amounts.

3. Pour the liquid mixture slowly into the dry mixture container in a way that it doesn't all fizz out all at once. Keep stirring while you pour.

4. Knead the solution to ensure the ingredients are completely combined together.

5. Put this mixture into the two halves of a bath bomb mold and press them together tightly.

6. Wait five minutes before removing the mold and let the bath bombs cure (harden) and dry for a day.

Tips and Tricks

---

1. Make sure you add the liquid ingredients one teaspoon at a time to avoid any sort of reaction when making the bath bomb.
2. Add the lemon zest to the mold's interior surface before pressing the rest of the mixture to give it an aesthetic look.

Floral Bath Bombs

Lavender

Lavender not only soothes your nerves and relieves stress but also moisturizes your skin, leaving it feeling fresh and smelling wonderful. This lavender recipe is made with skin-loving ingredients which will leave your skin feeling soft and scented after a bath. They're easy to prepare and don't require a lot of resources either.

Ingredients

- Baking soda – 1 cup or 128g
- Citric acid – ½ cup or 64g
- Cornstarch – ½ cup or 64g
- Epsom salts – ½ cup or 64g
- Fractionated coconut oil – 2 ½ cups or 320g
- Lavender buds – 2 tbsp
- Lavender essential oil – 10 drops
- Purple liquid coloring – 8 drops
- Water – As needed

Where to Find the Ingredients

You can easily find the main ingredients at any market near you. Lavender buds can be taken directly from its plant or bought separately. Epsom salts can be found at pharmacy stores or online.

Directions

1. Combine all the dry ingredients, i.e., baking soda, Epsom salts, citric acid, cornstarch, and dried lavender, together in a bowl and whisk them until completely mixed.

2. Ensure that you remove any lumps formed.

3. In a separate bowl, mix the essential oils, melted coconut oil, and water together.

4. Add the purple coloring to the liquid mix and stir.

5. Slowly pour the wet mixture into the dry mixture to ensure the reactive ingredients don't fizz out all at once.

6. Keep stirring as you add the liquid contents of the mixture into the dry ones until completely mixed.

7. Once they're mixed completely, take a small amount of the mixture into your hands, and squeeze it together to check to see if it holds its shape.

8. Press the mixture into the two halves of a bath bomb mold and shut them together tightly.

9. Remove the molds after ten minutes and leave the bath bombs to harden and dry for a day or two.

Tips and Tricks

1. To create a unique scent, add bergamot, sandalwood, and patchouli essential oils together and combine with lavender.
2. In case the bath bomb cracks when you're removing the mold, spray some water or witch hazel over it and press it back into the mold for five more minutes.

Ingredient Substitutions

Coconut oil	Almond oil
Essential Oils – lavender	Vanilla, chamomile

Rose

This all-natural floral bath bomb recipe contains rose petals, coconut oil, and a sweet blend of essential oils that will make your bath relaxing and nourishing. Rosewater is also used, which is very beneficial for your skin. Free of artificial dyes, these bath bombs will leave your skin feeling soft and supple.

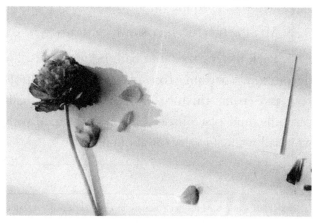

Ingredients

- Baking soda – 2 cups or 256g
- Citric acid – 1 ¼ cups or 160g
- Rose absolute – 70 drops or 3g
- Dried rose petals
- Pink pitaya powder – 1 tbsp
- Coconut oil – ⅓ cup or 80g
- Essential oil blend – 10g

Where to Find the Ingredients

You can easily find the main ingredients at any market near you. Pink pitaya powder can be found online. For the essential oil blend, you can use oils of your choice.

Directions

1. Let the coconut oil melt in a double boiler or microwave in one-minute intervals.

2. Let the melted oil cool off for around ten minutes before adding the essential oil blend and rose absolute.

3. Next, mix the citric acid with baking soda in a separate bowl. Add the dried rose petals to the mix.

4. Mix the two together slowly and stir.

5. Pack the mixture into bath bomb molds. For added decoration, put some rose petals inside the mold before you put your mixture in. Unmold the bath bomb carefully, and place it on a baking tray lined with bubble wrap, allowing it to dry for about a day.

Tips and Tricks

1. The petals can cause the bath bombs to crack or break; therefore, it is recommended to tear the petals into smaller pieces.
2. Wrap the bath bombs with plastic sheets or butter paper after drying.

Eucalyptus

Eucalyptus bath bombs are perfect for a relaxing bath to ease your sore muscles, and the Epsom salt in the mixture ensures that your tense muscles are eased. Plus, you can make these in any fragrance you like just by altering the essential oil blend a little. Peppermint and lavender usually work the best.

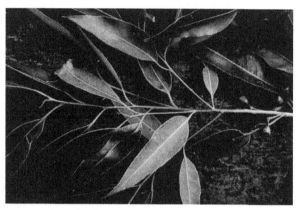

Ingredients

- Baking soda – 1 cup or 128g
- Citric acid – ½ cup or 64g
- Cornstarch – ½ cup or 64g
- Epsom Salts – ½ cup or 64g
- Almond oil – 3 tbsp
- Witch hazel – As needed
- Essential oil blend – 10g
- Soap coloring – 10 drops

Where to Find the Ingredients

Baking soda and citric acid can be found in your nearest grocery store. Epsom salts can be found online or in a pharmacy store. Soap coloring can be found online or in craft stores.

Directions

1. Mix the dry ingredients together and the wet ones in separate containers, making sure they are mixed thoroughly. Make sure you properly calculate the quantity of essential oils you add to your blend.

2. Add soap coloring to the liquid mix.

3. Combine the two mixtures together and whisk them together to fully incorporate the contents together.

4. Spritz the mixture with witch hazel and knead the mixture together.

5. Press the damp mixture into a bath bomb mold and let it dry for an hour.

6. Remove the mold and let the mixture dry further for a day or two.

Tips and Tricks
1. Make sure you add the liquid ingredients one teaspoon at a time to avoid any sort of reaction when making the bath bomb. 2. Place the bath bombs in an airtight container because exposure to moisture will make them foam prematurely.

Ingredient Substitutions	
Almond oil	Coconut oil
Witch hazel	Water
Epsom salt	Dead sea salts

Jasmine, Lily, and Aloe ★★★★☆

This recipe is a mix of jasmine flowers and aloe extracts, scented with white lily and aloe essential oils. The presence of aloe extracts makes it extremely beneficial for your skin and leaves it feeling soft and glowing.

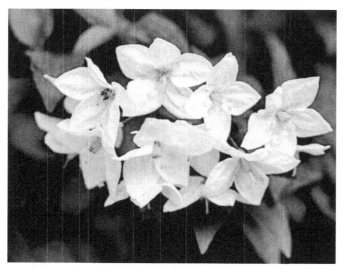

Ingredients

- Baking soda – 4 cups or 512g
- Citric acid – 2 cups or 256g
- Aloe extract – 1 oz. or 2 tbsp
- White lily and aloe fragrance oil – 1 tbsp
- Polysorbate 80 – 2 tsp
- Essential oil blend – 10g
- Witch hazel – As needed
- Jasmine flowers

Where to Find the Ingredients

You can easily find the main ingredients at any market near you. Jasmine flowers can be bought from a flower vendor or found online. You can extract aloe vera directly from its plant or buy it from the market.

Directions

1. Mix baking soda and citric acid together in a large bowl until thoroughly combined.

2. Add the essential oil blend with aloe extract and polysorbate in a jar, and shake well to mix them together.

3. Knead the two mixtures together to fully incorporate them together until you achieve a damp sand-like mixture.

4. Add a few jasmine flowers to the mold before throwing in the bath bomb mixture.

5. Press this mixture into bath bomb molds, ensure to create a high heap in the middle. Press the mold halves together tightly and wipe away any extra residue.

6. Unmold the bath bomb carefully, and place it on a baking tray lined with bubble wrap and allow it to dry for about a day.

Tips and Tricks

1. Make sure you add the liquid ingredients one teaspoon at a time to avoid any sort of reaction when making the bath bomb.
2. Extreme humidity can make it difficult to shape the bath bombs, so make sure to rehydrate the mixture with alcohol or witch hazel if you see it drying out when you put it into the mold.

Chapter 9: Foaming and Floaty Bath Bombs

One of the best things about bath bombs is their luscious bubbles in your bathwater. Fortunately, you can easily recreate this in homemade bath bombs. What's a little harder to produce is a floating bath bomb, as this property depends on a lot more factors than just the ingredients.

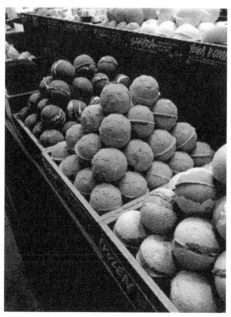

How Foaming Bath Bombs Are Made

The reaction between the acid and the base you use as the main ingredient already creates a certain degree of foam as it releases its byproduct, carbon dioxide. Now all you need is another ingredient to take the foaming to another level. One of the most popular ingredients to get added effect is SLSA or Sodium Lauryl Sulfoacetate. Derived from coconut or palm oil and sold in powdered form, SLSA can be found even in the commercially sold bath bombs. It's an organic product that also has gentle cleansing properties. The other ingredient which also helps to make more foam is milk powder. Made from dried milk, when it's soaked in water, milk powder is reconstituted, and if this happens in the middle of an acid-base reaction, the powder will foam profusely, and you get a super foamy bath bomb.

Aromatherapy Bath Bomb with Lavender

This recipe uses lavender essential oil, which has a very relaxing effect on your body and mind, alongside shea butter that will leave your skin soft and moisturized.

Ingredients

- Baking soda – 2 cups or 256g
- Citric acid – 1 1/4 cups or 160g
- Unrefined shea butter – 1/2 cup or 64g
- SLSA – ½ cup or 64 grams
- Lavender essential oil – 0.4 ounces or approximately 12 ml
- Witch hazel – as needed
- Mica powder in several colors – as needed
- Star sprinkles and glitter – optional for decoration

Where to Find the Ingredients

Most ingredients can be found in well-supplied supermarkets or health supply stores.

Directions

1. Melt the shea butter either in the microwave on the medium setting, and let it cool for 10 minutes afterward.

2. Once the shea butter has cooled, combine it with the lavender essential oil.

3. Slowly sift the citric acid and the baking soda in a large mixing bowl, then whisk in the SLSA as well.

4. Pour a little of the wet ingredients into the dry ones and start kneading the mixture immediately. Repeat until all the ingredients are combined.

5. Divide your mixture into separate containers, depending on how many colors you want to use.

6. Start adding the different colors of mica powder, sprinkle, and glitter into each partition until you are satisfied with the color.

7. Spray each batch with witch hazel, mix them, spritz them again, and then repeat the mixing until your formula reaches the consistency of wet sand. You should be able to mold the mixture into balls.

8. Once the mixture has reached the desired consistency, start transferring it into the molds. Doing it with your hands will help press down the mixture, so it forms a compact shape.

9. You can transfer the different colors into different molds or create multicolored bath bombs by alternating the colors into the same molds.

10. Once you have filled the molds, you can press two halves together to create whole shapes. Then take the

bomb out of the mold – tap the first half from the outside, then do the same with the other one.

11. Carefully place the bombs onto a tray and let them dry for about 1-2 days, depending on the humidity of your environment.

Tips and Tricks:
Transferring your mixture into the molds with your hands will help you press it down more to form a compact shape.

Substitutes:
You can substitute witch hazel with rubbing alcohol. You can also use mango butter instead of shea butter.

Warnings:
Don't use shea butter if you are allergic to nuts or shea in particular.

Milk and Honey Bath Bomb

The honey powder in this recipe has natural skin-tightening, anti-inflammatory, and antibacterial effects. Combined with the milk powder, honey can soothe irritated skin. Chamomile oil has very similar properties, while cocoa butter will serve as a deep moisturizing agent.

Ingredients

- Baking soda – 2 cups or 256g
- Citric acid – 1 1/4 cups or 160g
- Cocoa butter – ¾ cup or 96g
- Milk powder – ½ cup or 64g
- Honey powder – 0.9 ounces or 25 grams
- Chamomile essential oil up to 12 ml
- Yellow mica powder – 1 – 2 tsp or 5-10g

Where to Find the Ingredients

You will find the basic ingredients in convenient stores, whereas essential oils, cocoa butter, honey powder, and mica powder are sold in health and beauty supply stores.

Directions

1. Melt the cocoa butter in the microwave on the medium setting and let it cool for 10 minutes before adding the essential oil to it. If you want your bath bombs to be harder, you can add the polysorbate in this step as well.

2. Sift citric acid and baking soda into a large mixing bowl, then add the milk, honey, and mica powders to the mixture. Combine all these dry ingredients well.

3. Slowly start pouring the wet ingredients onto the dry ones, frequently stopping to knead the mixture.

4. Once the formula has reached a moldable consistency, start scooping it into the molds.

5. You will create half shapes and then press them together to form a whole.

6. After slowly unmolding the bombs, place them on a tray and leave them to dry for 24-48 hours, after which they will be ready to use.

7. Store the bath bombs in a cool place, and use them within a few weeks.

Tips and Tricks:
If you want your bath bombs to be harder, you can add polysorbate 80 in the first step as well.

Substitutes:
You can substitute cocoa butter with coconut oil.

Lime and Coconut Milk Bath Bomb

This recipe uses coconut milk powder, which has a nourishing effect, similar to hemp oil. Coconut milk is also a great alternative if you suffer from lactose sensitivity and can't use regular milk to make your bath bombs foam. The sea salt acts as an exfoliant, while the lime essential oil will have you revitalized after your bath.

Ingredients

- Baking soda - 2/3 cup or 153g
- Citric acid - 1/3 cup or 70g
- Cream of tartar - 1 1/2 tbsp or 15g
- Sea salt - 1 tbsp or 15g
- Coconut milk powder - 2 tbsp or 16g
- Hemp seed oil - 1 tbsp or 15 ml
- Lime essential oil - 20 drops 1 ml
- Witch hazel - as needed
- Liquid food coloring - as needed

Where to Find the Ingredients

Most ingredients for these recipes can be bought in health food stores or online.

Directions

1. In a large mixing bowl, combine citric acid, baking soda, coconut milk powder, cream of tartar, and sea salt. Make sure you mix these thoroughly by using your hands if needed.

2. Pour hemp seed oil and lime essential oil into another bowl and whisk them together.

3. Slowly add the liquid ingredients to the dry ones and mix them all together as quickly as you can.

4. Separate the mixture into a different container, according to the number of colors you are using. Add liquid food coloring to each batch.

5. Spray the mixture with a little bit of witch hazel, mix again, and check if it holds its shape. If it doesn't, spritz in a little more witch hazel.

6. Scoop the mixture into your mold and press it down with the back of your spoon or hand. If you are using half-spheres, press two of them together, then unmold the bombs.

7. Let your bath bombs dry for at least 12 hours, then check if they have solidified. If not, leave them for another 12 hours.

8. Use the bombs right away, or store them in airtight packaging for up to nine months.

Tips and Tricks:
If you are using molds made of metal, you can remove them easily by gently tapping them from outside with a spoon.

Substitutes:
Cream of tartar can be substituted with freshly squeezed lemon juice.

Mint Bath Bomb with Hidden Colors

The Epsom salts used in this recipe are great for muscle relaxation, while the mint oil will refresh your entire body and mind. The sweet almond oil is rich in vitamins and minerals needed by the skin to regain its healthy glow.

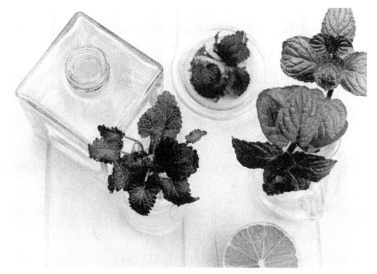

Ingredients

- Citric acid – 1 cup or 125g

- Baking soda – 2 cups or 250g

- Cornstarch – 1/2 cup or 60g

- Epsom salts – 1/2 cup or 56g

- Lake pigment – 1/4 tsp or 2g

- Mint essential oil – 20 drops or 1ml

- Sweet almond oil – 3 tbsp or 45ml

- Witch hazel – as needed

Where to Find the Ingredients

You can buy the ingredients for this recipe in pharmacies and beauty supply stores.

Directions

1. In one bowl, combine all the dry ingredients together, except the pigment.

2. Whisk the mint essential oil and sweet almond oil together in another bowl. Start adding the liquids slowly to the dry ingredients.

3. Mix all ingredients using your hands to feel the dryness of the formula.

4. Spray the mixture with witch hazel, mix again, then repeat the spritzing until it becomes moldable and holds its shape.

5. Place a good amount of the mixture in the half molds, add the pigment in the center of the half molds before pressing them together.

6. After unmolding them, put the bath bombs on a tray and leave them to dry for at least 24 hours.

Tips and Tricks:
Sealing the bath bombs after they dry will ensure that they stay dry and foam better when put in the water.

Substitutes:
You can substitute Epsom salts with Himalayan salt as it dissolves at the same speed.

Foaming Bath Bomb with Clay

This recipe uses Kaolin clay, which absorbs the excess oils on the skin, making it perfect to use on oily, problematic skin types. Jojoba oil also helps the skin look less shiny but more moisturized and more evenly colored at the same time.

Ingredients

- Baking soda - 1 cup or 250g
- Citric acid - 1/2 Cup or 100gr
- SLSA - 1 tbsp or 15g
- Kaolin clay - 1 tsp or 5g
- Cornstarch - 1/2 tbsp or 7.5g
- Jojoba oil - 1 tsp or 5 ml
- Polysorbate 80 - 1 tsp or 5g
- Fragrance (optional) - up to 15 drops or 0.7 ml
- Colored mica powder - 1 tbsp or 15g
- Water and alcohol Mixture (50:50) - as needed

Where to Find the Ingredients

You can buy baking soda, citric acid, and cornstarch in the local convenience store. The rest of the ingredients can be found in pharmacies.

Directions

1. Mix the polysorbate 80 with the colorant first to help disperse the pigment. Add this mixture to the other dry ingredients.

2. Combine jojoba oil and fragrance in another bowl, then start adding this into the dry mixture.

3. Mix all the ingredients with your hands, so you break up any clusters of dry ingredients.

4. Add in a couple of spritzes of the water and alcohol solution and continue to mix until you get a moldable mass.

5. Fill your half molds, press them together, and then carefully remove the molds from the bath bombs.

6. Place the bombs on the tray and wait for at least 24 hours before seeing if they are dry enough.

Tips and Tricks:
Because clay can cause the mixture to clump up, it's a good idea to mix everything with your hands so you can break up any clusters.

Substitutes:
You can substitute jojoba oil with avocado oil if you have dry skin.

How to Make Floating Bath Bombs

Whether your bath bombs will sink or float is determined by several factors. If a bath bomb is made with dense ingredients, it will be more likely to sink, whereas light, airy components will help it float. Flat-shaped bath bombs will stay on the surface longer than spherical ones, especially if they are molded correctly. The secret tip here is not to press your bath bombs as tightly as the others you've made because the air in them will help them stay afloat. In fact, you can even add a few air pockets manually as you press the mixture into the mold. You will also want to make sure your bath bombs are completely dry before using them. Otherwise, moisture will weigh them down, and they won't float.

Moisturizing Floating Bath Bomb

This recipe uses SLSA, which, apart from foaming, also gives a light texture to bath bombs. Coco betaine is another organic coconut derivative and has a similar effect, and it also moisturizes the skin. Frankincense essential oil has rejuvenating properties and will leave your skin tight and smooth.

Ingredients

- Citric acid – 2 cups or 250g
- Baking soda – 4 cups or 500g
- Coarse SLSA – 1 cup or 125g
- Frankincense essential oil – up to 20 drops or 1ml
- Liquid food coloring – as needed
- Cold water – 1/3 cup or approximately 80 ml
- Coco betaine – 1/4 teaspoon or 1ml

Where to Find the Ingredients

Most ingredients can be found in beauty supply stores or can be ordered online.

Directions

1. Combine citric acid, SLSA, and baking soda in a bowl and make sure everything is mixed thoroughly.

2. In another bowl, dissolve the food coloring in water, then add the Coco betaine to the water.

3. If you are using multiple colors, separate both the liquid and the dry ingredients into equal portions before adding each color.

4. Once your color is dissolved, you can slowly stir in the wet ingredients to the dry ones. Add the liquid in one tablespoon at a time.

5. Do each batch separately so you can mold them quickly after combining all ingredients?

6. When your mixture has reached the consistency of damp sand, you start adding it into your mold. Make your half mold, press together, and then unmold after a couple of seconds.

7. Place bath bombs on a tray and leave them to dry for 24-48 hours.

Tips and Tricks:

Don't overmix your bath bomb mixture because this will cause the air pockets to collapse and the formula to become denser.

Substitutes:

You can substitute frankincense essential oil with wild orange oil if you are looking for a more uplifting effect.

Easy Rainbow Bath Bomb

Because this recipe uses so few ingredients, there won't be too many things to weigh it down. While less potent than citric acid, lemon juice is also a great choice because it will slow the reaction time down, and your bath bomb will float for longer.

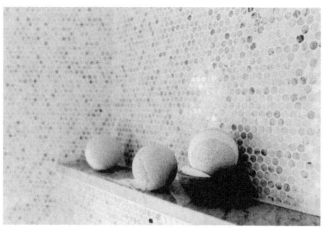

Ingredients

- Cornstarch – 1 tbsp or 15g
- Baking powder – 2 tbsp or 30g
- Lemon juice – 4 tsp or 20 ml
- Vanilla extract – 1 tsp or 5 ml
- Liquid food coloring – as needed

Where to Find the Ingredients

If you don't already have them in your pantry, you can get all ingredients at your local convenience store.

Directions

1. Mix the cornstarch and baking powder in one bowl and the lemon juice, vanilla extract in another one.

2. Combine the wet ingredients with the dry ones until everything is mixed well.

3. Separate into several batches and add different colors to each of them. This will also add essential moisture, so the mixture becomes malleable.

4. Scoop the mixture into your molds, layering the colors to create a rainbow effect.

5. After unmolding them, leave the bath bombs to dry for 24-48 hours and use them when needed.

Tips and Tricks:

While the mixture may seem dry initially, avoid adding water to it unless it's crumbling quite badly when trying to mold it. The liquid food coloring and the lemon juice should add essential moisture.

Substitutes:

You can substitute vanilla extract with any other edible-smelling aroma you have in your pantry.

Cookie Shaped Bath Bomb

Not only will these bath bombs smell delicious, but making them in small, flat cookie form will help them stay afloat longer. The grapeseed oils help moisturize the skin, while rosewood oil is safe to use on any skin type.

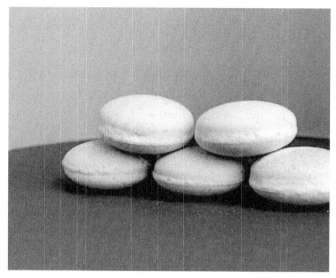

Ingredients

- Baking soda - 2 cups or 250g
- Citric acid - 1 cup or 125g
- Fine-grain salt - 1 cup or 125g
- Liquid food coloring - as needed
- Rosewood essential oil - 20 drops or 1 ml
- Water - as needed
- Grapeseed oil - 1/4 cup or approximately 60 ml

Where to Find the Ingredients

You may find rosewood essential oil in a pharmacy, while the rest of the ingredients are available in any supermarket.

Directions

1. Mix the dry ingredients in one bowl and the liquid ones in another one.

2. Combine everything together to make a uniform mixture and add as much food coloring as needed.

3. Continue mixing it with your hands while keeping a watch on the moldability of your formula. If it's too crumbly, spritz it with a little water.

4. Once the mixture can hold its form, scoop it up into cookie molds. As these already have a full shape, there won't be any need for further shaping.

5. Leave the bombs in the mold for 24 hours, then slowly get them out on a tray. Let them dry for another 48 hours, so they can be as floaty as possible.

Tips and Tricks:
After the initial 24 hours, let the bombs dry for at least another 48 hours before using them, so they can be as light as possible.

Substitutes:
You may substitute rosewood oil with lemon essential oil for a more lemon cookie scent.

Floral Scented Bath Bomb

The baby oil used in this recipe can work wonders on any skin type. It's also a lightweight oil, which means it won't weigh your bath bombs down. The floral fragrances create a lovely relaxing atmosphere and have a soothing effect on the skin.

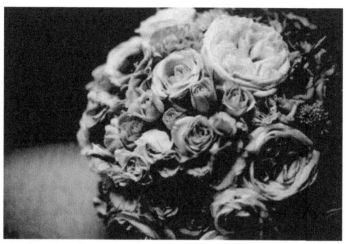

Ingredients

- Baking soda – 1 cup or 125g
- Citric acid – 1/2 cup or 65g
- Cornstarch – 1/2 cup or 65g
- Sea salt – 1/2 cup or 60g
- Water – 1 tbsp or 15 ml for each color
- Baby oil – 1 tbsp or 15 ml for each color
- Floral fragrance – 1 teaspoon or 5 ml for each color
- Liquid food coloring – 3-5 drops, or up to 0.25 ml

Where to Find the Ingredients

You can find all the ingredients in any convenience store or buy them in bulk online.

Directions

1. Mix citric acid, salt, baking soda, and cornstarch until well combined. Divide the mixture according to the number of colors you will use.

2. In several separate containers, combine fragrance, food coloring, water, and baby oil.

3. Slowly stir in the liquids to the dry ingredients by working with one batch at a time.

4. When you are done with one batch, scoop it into the molds. If you are making spheres, try to use the smallest ones possible, so your bath bombs wouldn't be too heavy.

5. Press the half spheres together, unmold after a couple of seconds, then place the bath bombs on a tray.

6. Once you are done with all your colors, let the bath bombs dry for at least 48 hours before placing them into an airtight container.

Tips and Tricks:
You can cut down the drying time by wrapping the bombs in cling film and dying them with a hairdryer.

Substitutes:
If your skin is too sensitive, you can substitute the baby oil with odorless mineral oil that is less likely to cause irritation.

Sparkly Floating Bath Bomb

This recipe uses rosehip oil which is another lightweight carrier oil. It's also fragrant on its own, so you can even leave out any additional essential oils or fragrances. The gentle formula is suitable for all skin types.

Ingredients

- Baking soda – 1 cup or 125g
- Cornstarch – 1/2 cup or 65g
- Citric acid – 1/2 cup or 65g
- Rosehip oil – 1 tsp or 5 ml
- Liquid food coloring – as needed
- Body glitter – as needed
- Water – as needed

Where to Find the Ingredients

Most of the ingredients will be available in health food stores or at a well-supplied supermarket.

Directions

1. Combine all the ingredients together, except the water and the food coloring.

2. Separate the mixture into three different bowls, and mix the food coloring into them. Do this one color at a time.

3. As soon as you have added color to a batch, start spraying it with water and kneading it continuously until you get a moldable mixture.

4. When you have mixed all your colors, fill two different half molds with two different colors. Leave a little space on top of them so you can add a small scoop of a third color. Press the molds together so the third color stays in the middle.

5. Unmold, then place on a tray to dry. Depending on how big the bath bombs are, they can take from 12 to 48 hours to dry.

Tips and Tricks:
Make sure you mix each batch as quickly as possible to avoid too much acid-base reaction during the preparation process.

Substitutes:
You can substitute liquid food coloring for mica powder and add a few more drops of water to make up for the lack of moisture.

Chapter 10: Storing, Packaging, and Labeling

This chapter explains how to store, package and label finished products. We take you through it step by step because if one step goes wrong – you'll find yourself having to remake your creations. You will also learn everything you need to know about the significance of packaging and labeling your products, particularly if you want to make it into a small business. The last part of the chapter focuses on product legislation.

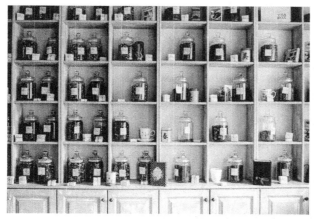

How to Store Bath Bombs

Bath bombs produce foam, and they will give you'll have the best experience if you use them while still fresh. If you do not use them on time, the ingredients will go bad. The other important point is about proper storage of your bath bombs because it is possible to use them long after making or buying them.

You need the appropriate containers for storage, and they must be stored in a dry and cool place to prevent issues like melting and fizzing. On average, your bath bombs can last up to six months if properly stored. To get this sort of shelf life, you must store all the bombs with the same ingredients in their own storage container. In other words, don't mix the different sorts of bath bombs together. They need to be kept separately. When the fragrances mix, their essence will be lost, which leaves you with useless bath bombs.

Get a non-porous container and also use a plastic bag to catch any crumbs (which you can also use in your bathtub). You should only keep the bath bomb in a storage container or wrap it after each use to prevent disintegration, but make sure you do this when it has dried completely. Another important safety tip is to keep your products away from direct sunlight or heat. When the bath bomb is exposed to heat, it will melt, and some of the ingredients will evaporate while the organic ones get damaged.

The golden rule is that you should store your bath bombs in a cool, dry place away from moisture and sunlight. No matter what type of products you have, you need to focus on good storage if you do not intend to use them immediately.

Packaging

To keep your bath bombs fresh for a long time, you should keep them in their own special containers. The following are some of the items you can use to store your products safely.

Bath Bomb Containers

Put the bath bomb in a special container designed for that purpose. Make sure you close the lid properly and put the container away from direct sunlight and heat. The other important thing to remember is that you must use an air-tight container to prevent any moisture from contaminating your bombs. Placing the container in a cool place helps prevent some ingredients, like essential oils and different kinds of body butter, from melting.

Use Plastic Wraps

Wrap your bath bombs tightly in plastic wrap, so they are not exposed to air. This preserves delicate fragrances and keeps your works of the art dry, and retains the quality and originality in general. Twist the end of the wrap, then tie a knot. You can use a sticker to seal off the knot and hide it, and if you have decorative stickers, it all adds to the beauty of the product you've made. You can also use a plastic bag, as long as you make sure all the air is out before you seal it.

Shrink Wraps

You can also use a shrink bag to store your bath bomb. When you use this, wrap the seal to ensure that it is air-tight. You can use a blower or hair dryer to blow some warm air on the bag to shrink it around the product inside. When you have completely sealed the bag, it should be stored in a cool, dry place.

Use Ziploc bags

You can also use Ziploc bags to store your bath bombs. Again, carefully make sure all the air is out of it before you zip it up. Keep the bag away from light or other heat sources.

Food Containers

If you don't have special packages to keep your bath bomb, you can use food containers or any other appropriate cans. Make sure you clean and dry them before storing your products in them. Check if the cans have lids since the products must be stored in an air-tight place. When using the bath bomb in the shower, take it out and close the container.

No matter what type of bath bombs you make, you can use any of the storage methods mentioned above. All you need to do is use air-tight containers, don't mix different types together, and keep them away from sunlight and other sources of heat. Packaging plays a crucial role in maintaining the quality and keeping your bombs safe. The other purpose of packaging is to appeal to potential customers. When you choose the right package and label for your product, this all goes toward making them attractive to buyers. The section below outlines in detail the significance of labeling the product packages.

Labeling

When you have found a suitable packaging for your bath bombs, now comes the time to label them if you intend to sell them or give them away as gifts. The significance of labeling products cannot be overstated, particularly in the retail environment. When consumers choose products to buy, they often evaluate the label, and this is the final step that will influence their decision-making process. The following are some of the main benefits of labeling each container.

Product Identification

The label on the product is the first thing that the customers will look at before they decide to buy. It can be called your first point of communication with your client and your chance to show off your professionalism and art. You can only recognize a brand or product through elements like a logo and the design. A distinct logo is one of the most identifiable features of a specific product. Labeling will help the consumer differentiate your product from all the others available on the market.

Labeling can also help to spread product awareness which means that it should be unique. Many people often only learn about a product when they come face to face with it on the shelves in retail stores. If the potential buyers are impressed by the product and how it looks and feels, you're halfway towards a sale and market awareness as they spread the word to their peers.

Strategic Marketing Tool

Labeling is a critical component for marketing a product to potential buyers. It helps to grab the attention of the customer who is looking for a specific product to solve their problems. Marketers use packaging and labeling to encourage consumers to try their products. With a proper label appealing to the right market, you can inform your users about how to use your product, as well as how to recycle or dispose of the container.

The most important thing about labeling is that it determines whether you will get the much-needed sale or not. When customers visit a shop, they know what they want to buy, but making a final decision can be overwhelming given the number of similar products available. This is where labeling comes in. It makes your product stand out from the rest. A label quickly conveys the uses offered by a particular product.

Your label should be colorful, bright, and well-designed to make your product visible among other offerings. However, your choice of colors and the overall design of your label should represent the "ambiance" of the type of product you are offering offers users. If it consists of natural ingredients, the label should also convey that same message to the customers. For instance, if you make organic bath bombs, your labeling should lean toward neutral colors.

The other opportunity labeling offers is that it gives you the chance to highlight the reasons why you think your product is better than others. If your bath bombs offer benefits, you should mention them. This information will compel the customer to try your product and investigate if the information provided is true. Many buyers are concerned about getting products that can solve their problems. Therefore, you must clearly state the reasons why you believe that your product is the best. Make sure the product provides an impression that will last.

Strengthening Brand Identity

Good packaging and labeling are critical to creating and reinforcing your brand identity. If consumers already know your brand and they like it, they are likely to choose it over other competing brand names. This, in turn, leads to brand loyalty, which is what you want, as this is what sustains and grows a business. Consistency in branding and theme helps the consumers find the goods they are familiar with. It also helps brand recognition, and many people can identify with it.

To strengthen your brand, consistency in colors and message is key to keeping your product differentiated from others. Your message must be clear and unambiguous and position your brand as a market leader in the industry. In this era of intense competition, you should make sure that your brand resonates with your clients and they keep coming back for more. All this can be achieved through using a properly researched labeling strategy.

Ingredients

A basic function of a label is to provide information about the product. All the different ingredients you've used must be spelled out clearly on the container or package for each different type of bath bomb. All the ingredients used in any product are clearly stated to help buyers know what they are purchasing. So, your details will help customers make informed decisions. And most importantly, you will be complying with the safety laws, which state that the buyer has the right to know the product's contents.

If a product contains any additives that can cause side effects, you need to include the details on the package. Cosmetic products like bath bombs can include chemical ingredients. You must display warning signs regarding the potential hazards and how to deal with them. All the information provided on the label must be correct, and you should not hide anything about your product. Some people are allergic to specific ingredients, and this means you should state clearly what the product is made of.

The other type of information that you need to include on the label concerns the manufacturing and expiry dates. Cosmetic products like bath bombs have life spans, so you must indicate the best before usage date on the label. When the product is past this date, it may not offer good results. In some instances, the products that have passed the expiry date can cause side effects. All these requirements protect you from losing customers and possibly avoiding potential lawsuits.

Instructions

Labeling also plays a vital role in providing instructions about how to use the product. If the product is used incorrectly, it can produce poor results and a bad experience. This can also have an impact on your product's performance in the market, especially if you get negative reviews. Some people can develop side effects if they fail to use a specific product in the right way.

To prove that your product is authentic, you should provide your contact details. You can include a website, e-mail address, telephone number, or physical address. This will help build loyalty if customers are able to contact you with their queries or even want to order custom-made products. You also need to respond to your customers promptly.

The instructions should also answer general questions such as e the time you may need to leave the product to take effect after use. It is essential to provide pertinent details about the storage of the product to help users get the best out of your product. This is particularly true for bath bombs for all the reasons stated about storage. There are regulatory bodies that provide guidelines for manufacturers of various products, which help them to meet standardized ways of presenting different details to consumers. When you are into the bath bomb-making business, make sure your labels include the following information.

- Ingredients
- Warnings
- Recipes
- Product use and care
- Product guarantees
- Weight statements
- Manufacture contact details
- Weight
- Best before date and expiration dates

Make sure you provide information that is easy to understand and avoid common mistakes that can confuse the users.

Bath Bombs Legislation

The other crucial aspect you should know about the bath bomb-making business concerns product legislation. Cosmetic products can be potentially harmful, so you need to meet the standard expectations. In each country, there is product legislation that provides important regulatory standards. This means that the manufacturers of cosmetic products are required by law to provide critical information such as ingredients and any usage warnings. In other words, a label is a legally required tag on items to inform the consumers about the products.

The other details you are compelled to provide on your packaging relate to the recycling of waste. You should ensure your container has a recycling logo displayed so that the customers know how to dispose of them safely. It's also eco-friendly and a point you can use in your marketing plans. The laws also compel the manufacturers to display contact details; as we stated above, consumers who might have issues with your product can easily contact you.

You should also display the number of contents to avoid short-changing the customers. In case of a hazardous product, you must provide a statutory warning as this is a legal requirement. The consumers must use the product with the full knowledge of its potential dangers so that they can make informed decisions. To avoid any legal issues, you must conduct further research – depending on your country – to provide necessary information to your customers. If you want to sell or gift the product, you should know the legal framework that guides your operations.

As you can see, storage, packaging, and labeling are critical components to understand if you want to succeed in your bath bomb-making business. It is essential to store your product in a cool, dry place, ensuring they retain their quality and also last a long time. Packaging comes in different forms, shapes, and sizes, so you must choose appropriate containers. Lastly, labeling is an effective marketing strategy that can influence the number of sales you can generate from your product. It also helps provide information about the bath bomb concerning its ingredients, instructions, and warning signs, if any.

Conclusion

The focus of this book was to introduce you to the magical world of bath bombs and explain how to make them at home. We have provided a number of recipes and explained the science behind the fizz. It informs the reader how bath bombs came to be and why they are important. The guide also explains why homemade organic bath bombs are a perfect choice – rather than buying commercially manufactured products.

Before you learn the art of crafting your own bath bombs at home, you'll have to gather some tools of the trade, learn a bit of the history, as well as reading some hints and tips. This practical DIY guidebook is unique in that it outlines instructions and steps to take when making these products. It explains the ingredients you need and how to use them at each stage of the process. Apart from ingredients, the guide also explains what tools you'll need and how to use them. The reader is also cautioned on what safety measures they should bear in mind when making bath bombs at home.

The main part of the book explains different components you should have, such as essential oils and other ingredients. It presents step-by-step instructions about how to measure and mix ingredients. Various scientific and chemical processes that take place at each stage are explained in detail to help the reader understand the different methods they can choose to customize their recipes.

The guide also provided tips about how to personalize the recipes and make the entire process fun and educational. In this book, you also learned different facets like making bath bombs for each type of skin, and we have included different recipes and ingredients. For instance, some recipes are specifically designed to soothe, de-stress, relax, as well as to calm the mind and skin. You also learned different measures you can take to experiment with new things when making bath bombs.

This book also explained critical things like storing, packaging, and labeling your finished bath bombs. It highlighted the significance of letting the product dry before use and also outlined the types of containers that can be used to store the product. Packaging and labeling play a pivotal role in marketing the product and making your product stand out from the rest. This guide provided you with all the tips that can make your final product attractive.

When you have mastered the art of making your bath bombs and are going to take your hobby to the next level, remember that all cosmetic products should meet expected standards before they hit the market. Likewise, it is imperative to understand different elements related to product legislation. The last part of the book presented crucial regulatory elements you should know about this kind of business. It provided tips about the measures you can take to avoid legal issues.

If you are ready to get started in this business, this workbook is for you. It explained everything you need to know about making your own natural and homemade bath bombs using simple recipes and organic ingredients.

Here's another book by Alice Burrell that you might like

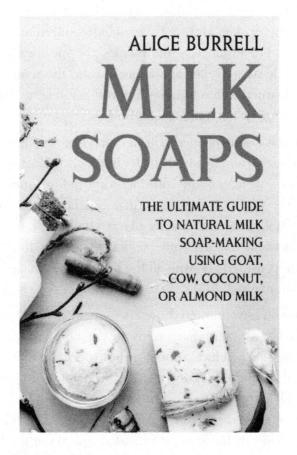

Resources

Are Bath Bombs Safe? (2019, August 21). Scripps.Org. https://www.scripps.org/news_items/6800-bath-bombs-are-they-safe

Hong, H. (2017, June 18). This is what's really in your bath bomb. Www.Rd.Com. https://www.rd.com/article/what-are-bath-bombs-made-of

Lush Fresh Handmade Cosmetics. (2019, August 22). A history of the bath bomb. Lushusa.Com; Lush Fresh Handmade Cosmetics. https://www.lushusa.com/stories/article-history-of-the-bath-bomb.html

Norris, R. (nod). Oh, this is how you're actually supposed to use a bath bomb. Byrdie.Com. Retrieved from https://www.byrdie.com/how-to-use-a-bath-bomb-4775435

Organic Bath Bombs and why they are so important for skin! (Nod). Bathbombbootcamp.Com. Retrieved from https://www.bathbombbootcamp.com/organic-bath-bombs.html

Segar, C. (2020, June 11). DIY bath bomb: Make bath bombs for every mood. OnlyMyHealth. https://www.onlymyhealth.com/diy-bath-bomb-make-bath-bombs-for-every-mood-1591878229

Zafar, S. (2021, July 6). How our skin benefits from the bath bombs. Bioenergyconsult.Com. https://www.bioenergyconsult.com/best-bath-bombs

7 benefits of kaolin clay & how to use it for skin. (2020, November 30). Skinkraft.Com. https://skinkraft.com/blogs/articles/kaolin-clay-for-skin

All-natural DIY bath bombs made the easy way. (2020, February 10). Gardentherapy.Ca. https://gardentherapy.ca/diy-bath-bombs

Bath Bomb Questions and Answers. (n.d.). Brambleberry.Com. Retrieved from https://www.brambleberry.com/ingredient-information/additives/art0001-bath-bomb-qa.html

Davidson, K., MScFN, RD, & CPT. (2020, October 14). 19 Household Uses for Cornstarch. Healthline.Com. https://www.healthline.com/nutrition/cornstarch-uses

DIY Craft Club. (n.d.). 5 reasons why your bath bombs are crumbling. Diycraftclub.Com. Retrieved from https://diycraftclub.com/blogs/idea-room-1/how-to-fix-crumbly-bath-bombs

Hamdani, S. (2021, February 17). 7 benefits of Witch Hazel for skin and way to use it. Bebeautiful.In; Be Beautiful India. https://www.bebeautiful.in/all-things-skin/everyday/benefits-of-witch-hazel-for-skin

Hannah. (2019, June 28). How to make DIY Lush Bath Bombs. Handmadeweekly.Com. https://www.handmadeweekly.com/diy-floral-bath-bombs

Heidi. (2016, October 14). DIY bath bombs: Where to find supplies plus tips and tricks.

Everydaysavvy.Com. https://everydaysavvy.com/diy-bath-bombs-find-supplies-plus-tips-tricks

Henry, E. (2018, November 2). DIY Donut Bath Bombs. Suburbansimplicity.Com.

https://www.suburbansimplicity.com/diy-donut-bath-bombs

hentis. (2019, November 22). How to make bath bombs harder? Strydomwebdevelopment.Co.Za.

https://strydomwebdevelopment.co.za/how-to-make-bath-bombs-harder

Hot to naturally color handmade soap. (n.d.). Bathbombbootcamp.Com. Retrieved from

https://www.bathbombbootcamp.com/naturally-color-handmade-soap.html

How to color bath bombs naturally? 10 simple steps. (2021, May 27). Nicegiftsnow.Com. https://nicegiftsnow.com/color-bath-bombs-naturally

How to make bath bombs – recipes and instructions for homemade bath bombs. (n.d.).

Homemade-Gifts-Made-Easy.Com. Retrieved from

https://www.homemade-gifts-made-easy.com/how-to-make-bath-bombs.html

Kauffman, A. (2019, September 23). How to make rainbow bath bombs at home.

Reallifeathome.Com. https://www.reallifeathome.com/how-to-make-rainbow-bath-bombs

Lewis, F. (2019, April 8). How to make bath bombs harder (3 easy tips). Showerplusbath.Com.

https://showerplusbath.com/how-to-make-bath-bombs-harder

Lobermeier, K. (2017, February 13). Herbal interests // 3 easy bath bomb recipes!

Underatinroof.Com; Under A Tin RoofTM.

https://www.underatinroof.com/blog/2017/2/17/herbal-interests-3-easy-bath-bomb-recipes

Nystul, J. (2020, December 26). DIY bath bomb recipe: How to make bath bombs at home. Onegoodthingbyjillee.Com.

https://www.onegoodthingbyjillee.com/how-to-make-your-own-lush-inspired-bath-bombs

Sarah. (2020, September 21). How to make DIY Bath Bombs. Feastforafraction.Com.

https://www.feastforafraction.com/diy-bath-bomb-recipe

Sehgal, K. (2021, April 29). 5 amazing benefits of essential Oils For Glowing Skin. NDTV

Swirlster. https://swirlster.ndtv.com/beauty/5-amazing-benefits-of-essential-oils-for-glowing-skin-2424440

Warren, V. A. P. by. (2020, October 29). The simple guide to coloring your bath bombs.

Daisysbeautyjewels.Com.

https://daisysbeautyjewels.com/2020/10/29/the-simple-guide-to-coloring-your-bath-bombs

(N.d.-a). Bathtubber.Com. Retrieved from

https://bathtubber.com/recommended-products/best-bath-bomb-supplies

(N.d.-b). Mindbodygreen.Com. Retrieved from

https://www.mindbodygreen.com/articles/diy-bath-bomb

(N.d.-c). Lifenreflection.Com. Retrieved from

https://www.lifenreflection.com/everything-you-need-to-make-bath-bombs

Quinn, D. (2021, February 17). Kaolin clay mask benefits for clearer, brighter skin.

Healthline.Com. https://www.healthline.com/health/beauty-skin-care/kaolin-clay-mask-benefits

5 major skin care benefits of roses. (2019, February 8). Skin Inc. https://www.skininc.com/science/ingredients/news/21887822/5-major-skin-care-benefits-of-roses

6 reasons to use lavender oil for skin. (n.d.). 100Percentpure.Com. Retrieved from

https://www.100percentpure.com/blogs/feed/6-reasons-to-use-lavender-oil-for-skin

8 surprising benefits of ylang essential oil. (2008, June 5). Organicfacts.Net.

https://www.organicfacts.net/health-benefits/essential-oils/health-benefits-of-ylang-ylang-essential-oil.html

10 beauty benefits of turmeric essential oil. (2020, April 23).

13 wonderful benefits of Cedarwood essential oil. (2008, April 7). Organicfacts.Net.

https://www.organicfacts.net/health-benefits/essential-oils/health-benefits-of-cedar-wood-essential-oil.html

15 uses and benefits of frankincense essential oil. (2020, September 11). Ilavahemp.Com. https://ilavahemp.com/frankincense-essential-oil

20 incredible health benefits of eucalyptus oil that seem too good to be true. (n.d.).

Sonomalavender.Com. Retrieved from https://www.sonomalavender.com/blogs/news/20-incredible-health-benefits-of-eucalyptus-oil

Are essential oils safe? (n.d.). Umn.Edu. Retrieved from

https://www.takingcharge.csh.umn.edu/are-essential-oils-safe

Axe, J., DC, DNM, & CN. (2018, November 28). Lemongrass essential oil uses & benefits, for skin, hair & more – Dr. Axe. Draxe.Com. https://draxe.com/essential-oils/lemongrass-essential-oil

Benefits of Rose oil and its side effects. (2017, October 6). Lybrate.Com.

https://www.lybrate.com/topic/benefits-of-rose-oil-and-its-side-effects

Choudhary, T. (2014, May 23). 15 amazing benefits of chamomile oil for skin, health, and hair. Stylecraze.Com; StyleCraze.

https://www.stylecraze.com/articles/amazing-benefits-of-chamomile-oil-for-skin-health-and-hair

Eucalyptus: Uses, side effects, interactions, dosage, and warning. (n.d.). Webmd.Com. Retrieved from https://www.webmd.com/vitamins/ai/ingredientmono-700/eucalyptus

GR. (2020, December 7). Bath bombs with essential oils: Ultimate DIY guide.

Everlastingcomfort.Net. https://www.everlastingcomfort.net/blogs/comfy-reads/how-to-make-bath-bombs-with-essential-oils

Helen West, R. D. (2019, September 30). What are essential oils, and do they work?

Healthline.Com. https://www.healthline.com/nutrition/what-are-essential-oils

How much Essential oils should I used with various age groups? (n.d.). Birchhillhappenings.Net. Retrieved from https://birchhillhappenings.net/safe-amounts-to-use.html

Isabella. (2020, August 11). 10 benefits of tea Tree essential oil for skin, hair, and health — isabella's clearly. Isabellasclearly.Com; Isabella's Clearly.

https://www.isabellasclearly.com/blog/10-benefits-of-tea-tree-essential-oil

Joanna. (2018, August 17). The benefits of essential oils in bath bombs. Jojotastic.Com. https://jojotastic.com/2018/08/17/essential-oil-bath-bomb-benefits

Johnson, J. (2019, October 18). What are essential oils? Uses and side effects.

Medicalnewstoday.Com. https://www.medicalnewstoday.com/articles/326732

Knight, D. (n.d.). 5 skincare benefits of chamomile (and 8 products to try). Byrdie.Com. Retrieved from https://www.byrdie.com/skincare-benefits-of-chamomile-4691698

Krouse, L. (2020, February 3). 7 genius ways eucalyptus oil can benefit your health, according to experts. Prevention.Com; Prevention.

 https://www.prevention.com/health/a30615989/eucalyptus-oil-benefits

Lemongrass: Uses, side effects, interactions, dosage, and warning. (n.d.). Webmd.Com.

Retrieved from https://www.webmd.com/vitamins/ai/ingredientmono-719/lemongrass

Lidicker, G., & S., M. (2019, September 30). The essential oils you should never put in your bath. Mindbodygreen.Com; mindbodygreen. https://www.mindbodygreen.com/articles/which-essential-oils-are-safe-for-bathtub

Petre, A., MS, & (nl), R. D. (2021, March 9). 5 benefits and uses of frankincense — and 7 myths. Healthline.Com. https://www.healthline.com/nutrition/frankincense

Sehgal, K. (2021, April 29). 5 amazing benefits of essential Oils For Glowing Skin. NDTV

Swirlster. https://swirlster.ndtv.com/beauty/5-amazing-benefits-of-essential-oils-for-glowing-skin-2424440

Seladi-Schulman, J. (2019, August 14). The 8 proven benefits of chamomile oil and how to use it. Healthline.Com. https://www.healthline.com/health/chamomile-oil

Tadimalla, R. T. (2015, April 29). 11 benefits and uses of ylang essential oil for health, skin,

hair. Stylecraze.Com; StyleCraze. https://www.stylecraze.com/articles/benefits-of-ylang-ylang-oil

Turmeric. (n.d.). Rxlist.Com. Retrieved from https://www.rxlist.com/turmeric/supplements.htm

What is the difference between carrier oil and essential oil. (2020, July 9). Pediaa.Com.

https://pediaa.com/what-is-the-difference-between-carrier-oil-and-essential-oil

What to know about Cedarwood essential oil. (n.d.). Webmd.Com. Retrieved from

https://www.webmd.com/balance/what-to-know-about-cedarwood-essential-oil

Whelan, C. (2020, February 10). Ylang essential oil uses & benefits. Healthline.Com.

https://www.healthline.com/health/ylang-ylang

Wong, C. (n.d.-a). Essential Oils for Stress Relief. Verywellmind.Com. Retrieved from

https://www.verywellmind.com/essential-oils-to-help-ease-stress-89636

Wong, C. (n.d.-b). The health benefits of lavender essential oil. Verywellmind.Com. Retrieved

from https://www.verywellmind.com/lavender-for-less-anxiety-3571767

Wong, C. (n.d.-c). What is chamomile? Verywellhealth.Com. Retrieved from

https://www.verywellhealth.com/the-benefits-of-chamomile-89436

Zee, M. (n.d.). 15 ways you can use tea tree oil. Byrdie.Com. Retrieved from

https://www.byrdie.com/uses-for-tea-tree-oil-5079155

(N.d.). Bathtubber.Com. Retrieved from https://bathtubber.com/10-best-essential-oils-for-bath-bombs

Beckwith, R. (n.d.). How to make a bath bomb. Retrieved from Bbcgoodfood.com website: https://www.bbcgoodfood.com/howto/guide/how-make-bath-bomb

(N.d.). Retrieved from Scientificamerican.com website:

https://www.scientificamerican.com/article/sudsy-science-creating-homemade-bath-bombs

Rowan, K. (2018, December 22). The science of bath bombs (and how to make them). Retrieved from Live Science website: https://www.livescience.com/64381-how-to-make-bath-bombs.html

Are bath bombs safe for children? (2019, November 4). Retrieved from Jewelwithin.com website: https://www.jewelwithin.com/are-bath-bombs-safe-for-children

Are bath bombs safe for toddlers what you need to know. (2021, March 6). Retrieved from Bath-ritual.com website: https://bath-ritual.com/are-bath-bombs-safe-for-toddlers

Ashley at Frugal Coupon Living. (2020, April 13). Homemade kids Bath Bombs – you choose the scent! Retrieved from Frugalcouponliving.com website:

https://www.frugalcouponliving.com/homemade-kids-bath-bombs

Bath bomb recipe for kids. (2020, May 15). Retrieved from Thebestideasforkids.com website: https://www.thebestideasforkids.com/bath-bomb-recipe-for-kids

Crystal. (2016, November 2). How to make DIY bath bombs with A toy hidden inside. Retrieved from Hellocreativefamily.com website: https://hellocreativefamily.com/how-to-make-diy-bath-bombs-with-a-toy-hidden-inside

Freydkin, D. (2019, April 18). The best bath bombs for kids to get their fizz on. Retrieved from Fatherly.com website: https://www.fatherly.com/gear/best-bath-bombs-for-girls-and-boys

Irena. (2019, July 25). Homemade bath bombs without citric acid – bath bomb recipe for kids. Retrieved from Countryhillcottage.com website: https://www.countryhillcottage.com/bath-bombs-without-citric-acid

Musti. (2021, March 10). Are bath bombs safe for kids? Retrieved from Diyproducts101.com website: https://www.diyproducts101.com/are-bath-bombs-safe-for-kids

Soken-Huberty, E. (2020, April 25). 10 reasons why family is important. Retrieved from Theimportantsite.com website: https://theimportantsite.com/10-reasons-family-is-important

Thatcher, T. (2020, March 17). The top ten benefits of spending time with family. Retrieved from Highlandspringsclinic.org website: https://highlandspringsclinic.org/blog/the-top-ten-benefits-of-spending-time-with-family

Bramble Berry. (2018, December 28). Relaxing Lavender Bath Bombs – soap queen. Retrieved

from Soapqueen.com website:

https://www.soapqueen.com/bath-and-body-tutorials/relaxing-lavender-bath-bombs

Busick, J. (2019, January 9). How bath bombs blow away your stress. Retrieved from

Soapboxsoaps.com website:

https://www.soapboxsoaps.com/blogs/soapbox-blog/how-bath-bombs-blow-away-your-stress

Clarabut, J. (2019, April 15). Why relaxation is so important. Retrieved from

Wellbeingpeople.com website:
https://www.wellbeingpeople.com/2019/04/15/why-relaxation-is-so-important

Derrick, J. (n.d.). Relax, soothe, and save money with this DIY bath bomb recipe. Retrieved

from Byrdie.com website: https://www.byrdie.com/basic-bath-bomb-recipe-346761

fitasamamabear. (2017, October 14). DIY sleepy time bath bombs with essential oils to promote relaxation. Retrieved from Fitasamamabear.com website:

https://fitasamamabear.com/diy-sleepy-time-bath-bombs

fitasamamabear. (2018, March 24). Stress relief DIY bath bombs-made with essential oils.

Retrieved from Fitasamamabear.com website:
https://fitasamamabear.com/diy-stress-relief-bath-bombs

Rina. (2017, December 17). Meditation Bath Bomb Recipe – the most relaxed you'll ever feel! –

sweet nature's beauty. Retrieved from Sweetnaturesbeauty.com website:

https://sweetnaturesbeauty.com/meditation-bath-bomb-recipe

White, D. M., LMHC, & CACP. (2016, May 17). Relaxation: Make time and take time for self-care. Retrieved from Psychcentral.com website:

https://psychcentral.com/lib/relaxation-make-time-and-take-time-for-self-care

Affeld, M. (2021, March 26). 7 DIY bath bombs for a soothing, relaxing soak. Insteading.Com.

https://insteading.com/blog/diy-bath-bombs

Derrick, J. (n.d.). Relax, soothe, and save money with this DIY bath bomb recipe. Byrdie.Com.

Retrieved from https://www.byrdie.com/basic-bath-bomb-recipe-346761

DIY moisturizing bath bombs to soothe dry, winter skin. (2016, January 31). Goodlifeeats.Com. https://www.goodlifeeats.com/diy-moisturizing-bath-bombs

Easy bath bomb recipe with natural ingredients for beautiful glowing skin. (2019, July 15). Soapdelinews.Com.

https://soapdelinews.com/2019/07/easy-bath-bomb-recipe-natural-ingredients-beautiful-glowing-skin.html

Griffis, T. (2021, June 8). Ultra-hydrating coconut bath bombs {easy DIY}.

Livingwellmom.Com. https://livingwellmom.com/coconut-bath-bombs

Irena. (2019, June 25). DIY moisturising bath bombs recipe – homemade milk & honey bath bombs. Countryhillcottage.Com.

https://www.countryhillcottage.com/diy-moisturising-bath-bombs-recipe

Olay UK. (2020, August 3). What is my skin type – Oily, dry, or mixed; what is the difference?

Olay.Co.Uk; Olay UK. https://olay.co.uk/skin-care-tips/oily-skin/find-out-your-skin-type

Sarah. (2020, September 21). How to make DIY Bath Bombs. Feastforafraction.Com.

https://www.feastforafraction.com/diy-bath-bomb-recipe

(N.d.). Lifenreflection.Com. Retrieved from
https://www.lifenreflection.com/oatmeal-bath-bomb-recipe

Charlene. (2017, January 26). Eucalyptus Bath Bombs.
Myfrugaladventures.Com.

https://myfrugaladventures.com/2017/01/eucalyptus-bath-bombs

Forest Berries Fruit Tea Bath Bombs Recipe – easy DIY. (2019,
August 7).

Consumerqueen.Com. https://consumerqueen.com/diy-projects-
2/fruit-tea-bath-bombs

Formaro, A. (2021, February 5). Lavender bath bombs.
Craftsbyamanda.Com.

https://craftsbyamanda.com/lavender-bath-bombs

Irena. (2020, June 10). How to make Rose petal bath bombs
{natural + moisturizing recipe}. Countryhillcottage.Com.
https://www.countryhillcottage.com/diy-rose-petal-bath-bombs

Laura. (2021, July 13). Homemade tropical bath bombs.
Ouroilyhouse.Com.

https://www.ouroilyhouse.com/homemade-tropical-bath-bombs

Lily and Aloe Bath Bomb Project. (n.d.). Brambleberry.Com.
Retrieved from

https://www.brambleberry.com/in-the-studio/projects/bath-
bombs/lily-and-aloe-bath-bomb-project/PS000075.html

Nicole. (2020a, May 6). Lemon Vanilla bath bomb recipe.
Momalwaysfindsout.Com.

https://www.momalwaysfindsout.com/recipe/lemon-vanilla-bath-
bomb-recipe

Nicole. (2020b, August 6). How To Make Bath Bombs.
Momalwaysfindsout.Com.

https://www.momalwaysfindsout.com/recipe/strawberry-bath-
bomb-recipe

ChrisW. (2021, May 10). How to store bath bombs: Bath bomb storage ideas. Retrieved from

Highshower.com website: https://highshower.com/store-bath-bombs

Admin, C. T. M. (2020, September 14). The importance of product labeling. Retrieved from Ctmlabelingsystems.com website: https://ctmlabelingsystems.com/labeling/the-importance-of-product-labeling

Sharma, K. (2015, January 22). Importance of Labelling. Retrieved from

Packagingconnections.com website:

https://www.packagingconnections.com/blog-entry/importance-labelling.htm

Bomb Guru. (2020, December 8). (answered) should bath bombs float or sink? Retrieved from Bathbombguide.com website: https://bathbombguide.com/should-bath-bombs-float-or-sink

Irena. (2019, July 3). DIY foaming bath bombs with Shea butter – aromatherapy bath bombs for

sleep & relaxation. Retrieved from Countryhillcottage.com website:

https://www.countryhillcottage.com/aromatherapy-bath-bombs-for-sleep-relaxation-diy-foaming-bath-bombs-with-shea-butter

Irena. (2019a, June 25). DIY moisturising bath bombs recipe – homemade milk & honey bath

bombs. Retrieved from Countryhillcottage.com website:

https://www.countryhillcottage.com/diy-moisturising-bath-bombs-recipe

The best fizzing & spinning DIY bath bomb recipe. (2021, February 24). Retrieved from Diynatural.com website: https://www.diynatural.com/spinning-bath-bomb-recipe

Jane, Clarice, Tisha, Macy, Shirley, & Nancy. (2018, August 22). Make a Bath Bomb float like LUSH. Retrieved from Howtobathbombs.com website:

http://howtobathbombs.com/wp/2018/08/22/make-a-bath-bomb-float-like-lush

Can't miss recipe for foaming bath bombs. (n.d.). Retrieved from Rntozen.com website: https://www.rntozen.com/foaming-bath-bomb-recipe

11 benefits of using natural body butter. (n.d.). Magical-Tree.Com. Retrieved from

https://www.magical-tree.com/blogs/our-story/11-benefits-of-using-natural-body-butters

All about Shea Butter: History & benefits. (2016, August 24). Bettersheabutter.Com.

https://bettersheabutter.com/about-us/benefits-shea-butter

Benefits of body butter. (n.d.). Oliviasheritage.Com. Retrieved from

https://oliviasheritage.com/blogs/news/benefits-of-body-butter

Bharat, D. (2021, August 10). Body butter: Splendid benefits to soothe dry skin and the different

types. Netmeds. https://www.netmeds.com/health-library/post/body-butter-splendid-benefits-to-soothe-dry-skin-and-the-different-types

Body lotion vs. body butter: Which works best for your skin type? (2020, January 11).

Healthshots.Com. https://www.healthshots.com/beauty/skin-care/body-lotion-vs-body-butter-which-works-best-for-your-skin-type

Botaneri, D. @. (2018, November 12). 6 reasons homemade skincare is more effective than big brands. Botaneri.Com. https://botaneri.com/6-reasons-homemade-skincare-effective

Castro, M. (2020, January 1). The benefits of homemade natural Body Butter.

Migiceracandles.Com; Migi Cera Candle Co. https://migiceracandles.com/blogs/migi-blog/the-benefits-of-homemade-natural-body-butter

Cocoa Butter - benefits & uses for ultimate skin care & personal care. (n.d.).

Newdirectionsaromatics.Com. Retrieved from

https://www.newdirectionsaromatics.com/blog/products/all-about-cocoa-butters.html

Copyright © Kao Corporation. All rights reserved. (n.d.). What is body butter? Jergens.Com.

Retrieved from https://www.jergens.com/en-us/blog/healthy-skin/what-is-body-butter

Debczak, M. (2016, March 23). Shea butter was first made 1000 years earlier than previously

thought. Mentalfloss.Com. https://www.mentalfloss.com/article/77627/shea-butter-was-first-made-1000-years-earlier-previously-thought

Debutify, & Sublime Life. (2020, October 20). Body lotion vs. Body Butter vs. Body Oil: Which

one is right for me? Sublimelife.In. https://sublimelife.in/blogs/sublime-stories/difference-between-body-butters-oils-and-lotions

Everything you need to know about body butter. (n.d.). Ilovecosmetics.Co.Uk. Retrieved from

https://www.ilovecosmetics.co.uk/blog/everything-you-need-to-know-about-body-butter

Origins of Shea Butter. Fascinating Benefits of Shea butter for hair and skin. (2019, February

28). Naturallivingsupplies.Co.Uk. https://naturallivingsupplies.co.uk/shea-butter-history-and-benefits

Werner, A. (2019, September 24). Commonly overlooked benefits of Body Butter.

Whishbody.Com. https://whishbody.com/blogs/news/body-butter-benefits

What is Body Butter? (n.d.). Thebodyshop.Com. Retrieved from

https://www.thebodyshop.com/en-gb/tips-and-advice/what-is-body-butter/e/e00057

(N.d.). Researchgate.Net. Retrieved from

https://www.researchgate.net/publication/275968288_The_Evolution_of_Shea_Butter's_Paradox_of_paradoxa_and_the_Potential_Opportunity_for_Information_and_Communication_Technology_ICT_to_Improve_Quality_Market_Access_and_Women's_Livelihoods_across_Rural_

Aromatherapist, J. L.-C. (2018, April 19). How to whip Shea butter without heat - DIY essential

oil recipes. Lovingessentialoils.Com. https://www.lovingessentialoils.com/blogs/diy-recipes/how-to-whip-shea-butter-without-heat

Grey, C. (n.d.). How to temper cocoa butter for making products. Camdengrey.Com. Retrieved

from https://www.camdengrey.com/blog/how-to-temper-cocoa-butter-for-making-products

How to make whipped Body Butters. (2013, February 20). Naturalbeautyworkshop.Com.

https://naturalbeautyworkshop.com/my_weblog/2013/02/how-to-make-whipped-body-butters-1.html?doing_wp_cron=1638197925.0093901157379150390625

How to use essential oils in body butter. (2018, July 13). Artsyfartsylife.Com.

https://artsyfartsylife.com/how-to-use-essential-oils-in-body-butters

Isabella. (2018, September 21). How to make whipped Shea butter? Melted or cold?

Bettersheabutter.Com. https://bettersheabutter.com/how-to-whip-shea-butter-melt-whip-or-cold-whip

11 surprising benefits of chamomile essential oil. (2008, April 5). Organicfacts.Net.

https://www.organicfacts.net/health-benefits/essential-oils/camomile-essential-oil.html

Allen, M. (2021, November 5). 15 beauty benefits of lavender oil that'll make you a believer.

The Thirty. https://thethirty.whowhatwear.com/benefits-of-lavender-oil/slide25

Cherney, K. (2019, July 8). 23 essential oils for skin conditions and types, and how to use them.

Healthline.Com. https://www.healthline.com/health/essential-oils-for-skin

Clary sage essential oil. (n.d.). Decleor.Com. Retrieved from https://www.decleor.com/en/oil-effects/draining/clary-sage.html

Geranium essential oil / Geranium bourbon essential oil. (n.d.). Decleor.Com. Retrieved from

https://www.decleor.com/en/oil-effects/cell-stimulation/geranium.html

How to use essential oils in body butter. (2018, July 13). Artsyfartsylife.Com.

https://artsyfartsylife.com/how-to-use-essential-oils-in-body-butters

Isabella. (2017, March 6). Essential oils for skin care recipes. Bettersheabutter.Com.

https://bettersheabutter.com/how-to-add-essential-oils-in-your-homemade-skin-care-products

Neroli essential oil. (n.d.). Decleor.Com. Retrieved from
https://www.decleor.com/en/oil-effects/moisture-lock/neroli.html

Our essential oils. (n.d.). Decleor.Com. Retrieved from
https://www.decleor.com/en/our-essential-oils

Rosemary essential oil. (n.d.). Decleor.Com. Retrieved from
https://www.decleor.com/en/oil-effects/antibacterial/rosemary-47.html

Sandalwood essential oil. (n.d.). Decleor.Com. Retrieved from
https://www.decleor.com/en/oil-effects/moisture-lock/sandalwood.html

Schaefer, A. (2021, July 14). Sandalwood oil: Health benefits and uses. Healthline.Com.
https://www.healthline.com/health/what-is-sandalwood

Seladi-Schulman, J. (2019, August 14). The 8 proven benefits of chamomile oil and how to use
it. Healthline.Com.
https://www.healthline.com/health/chamomile-oil

Taylor, S. (2018, August 13). How to make homemade whipped body butter using essential oils.

Bellatory. https://bellatory.com/skin/Homemade-Body-Butter-Recipe-Using-Essential-Oils

Tea Tree Essential Oil for skincare: history, benefits, and use – Decléor UK. (n.d.).

Decleor.Com. Retrieved from https://www.decleor.com/en/oil-effects/antibacterial/tea-tree.html

The health potential of Rosemary. (2014, November 14). Healthline.Com.

https://www.healthline.com/health/rosemary-health-potential

Whelan, C. (2017, June 20). Clary sage: Benefits and uses of this essential oil. Healthline.Com.

https://www.healthline.com/health/clary-sage

(N.d.). Doterra.Com. Retrieved from https://www.doterra.com/US/en/blog/spotlight-lavender-oil

Cabanel, E. (2014, March 30). Shea body butter recipe. Organic-Beauty-Recipes.Com.

https://www.organic-beauty-recipes.com/shea-body-butter-recipe

Cabanel, E. (2017a, July 1). Coconut oil body butter recipe like body shop but without the

chemicals. Organic-Beauty-Recipes.Com.

https://www.organic-beauty-recipes.com/coconut-oil-body-butter-recipe

Cabanel, E. (2017b, August 12). Mango body butter recipe. Organic-Beauty-Recipes.Com.

https://www.organic-beauty-recipes.com/mango-body-butter-recipe

Cabanel, E. (2017c, October 20). Ucuuba body butter recipe. Organic-Beauty-Recipes.Com.

https://www.organic-beauty-recipes.com/ucuuba-butter-body-recipe

Cabanel, E. (2020, July 12). DIY whipped body butter. Organic-Beauty-Recipes.Com.

https://www.organic-beauty-recipes.com/diy-whipped-body-butter

Decadent DIY whipped argan oil body butter recipe. (n.d.). Mystrikingly.Com. Retrieved from

https://arganoilproductreviews.mystrikingly.com/blog/diy-whipped-argan-oil-body-butter-recipe

Gamble, L. (2020, January 3). Natural vanilla body butter recipe. Momprepares.Com. https://momprepares.com/vanilla-body-butter

Handmade honey body butter recipe for radiant skin. (2021, January 21). Lovelygreens.Com.

https://lovelygreens.com/honey-body-butter-recipe

Jones, O. (2018, April 13). Argan oil for body. Arganoilproductreviews.Com; Argan Oil Product

Reviews. https://www.arganoilproductreviews.com/skin-care/body

Tiffany-The Coconut Mama. (2015, November 28). Easy DIY whipped body butter (only 4

ingredients). Thecoconutmama.Com.

https://thecoconutmama.com/homemade-body-butter

(N.d.). Simplelifemom.Com. Retrieved from

https://simplelifemom.com/2020/07/20/chamomile-body-butter-recipe

Babassu oil: Are there health benefits? (n.d.). Webmd.Com. Retrieved from

https://www.webmd.com/diet/babassu-oil-health-benefits

Citrus fresh body butter. (2015, May 16). Totallythebomb.Com.

https://totallythebomb.com/citrus-fresh-body-butter

Eghbali, E. (2015, November 3). How to make a body butter. Formulabotanica.Com.

https://formulabotanica.com/how-to-make-a-body-butter

Handmade honey body butter recipe for radiant skin. (2021, January 21). Lovelygreens.Com.

https://lovelygreens.com/honey-body-butter-recipe

How to use and make Comfrey Oil (and why it is controversial). (2019, June 15).

Lovelygreens.Com. https://lovelygreens.com/how-to-make-comfrey-oil-controversial

Lampman, E. (2014, December 17). DIY Gingerbread Body Butter. Frugalmomeh.Com.

https://www.frugalmomeh.com/diy-gingerbread-body-butter.html

Margarita. (2021a, October 6). How to make turmeric-infused oil for skin [7 easy steps].

Diybeautybase.Com. https://diybeautybase.com/how-to-make-turmeric-infused-oil

Margarita. (2021b, October 7). Brightening turmeric body butter recipe. Diybeautybase.Com.

https://diybeautybase.com/turmeric-body-butter-recipe

Scaccia, A. (2017, January 17). Avocado oil for skin: Benefits, use, and more. Healthline.Com.

https://www.healthline.com/health/beauty-skin-care/avocado-oil-for-skin

Sweet & Spicy whipped body butter. (n.d.). Thearomatherapist.Com. Retrieved from

https://www.thearomatherapist.com/blogs/recipes/diy-sweet-spicy-whipped-body-butter

The complete list of essential oil substitutes (80+ oils listed!). (n.d.). Sacredsoulholistics.Co.Uk.

Retrieved from https://www.sacredsoulholistics.co.uk/blogs/news/essential-oil-substitutes

11 benefits of using natural body butter. (n.d.). Magical-Tree.Com. Retrieved from

https://www.magical-tree.com/blogs/our-story/11-benefits-of-using-natural-body-butters

Anti-cellulite smoothing whipped body butter. (2019, August 28). Greenthickies.Com.

https://www.greenthickies.com/anti-cellulite-smoothing-whipped-body-butter

Claire, C. @. C., Therapeutic Aesthetics, Holidays, F., Collins, C., Bree, suptosarkar, & Mannu.

(2019, March 1). DIY Shea Butter Hair Conditioner Recipe. Theurbanumbrella.Com. https://www.theurbanumbrella.com/diy-shea-butter-hair-conditioner-recipe

Colleen. (2018, October 31). Dry skin whipped body butter recipe. Howbeautifullifeis.Com. https://howbeautifullifeis.com/moisturising-anti-ageing-whipped-body-butter-recipe-for-very-dry-skin

DIY cleansing balm to melt your makeup. (2017, March 24). Alifeadjacent.Com. https://alifeadjacent.com/makeup-melting-cleansing-balm

Mamta. (2017, August 27). DIY anti-itch whipped body butter for eczema-prone skin. Alluringsoul.Com. https://alluringsoul.com/diy-whipped-body-butter-for-eczema-prone-skin

Maura. (2021, March 10). DIY cuticle softener. Livingwellmom.Com. https://livingwellmom.com/homemade-cuticle-butter

Tiffany-The Coconut Mama. (2015, November 28). Easy DIY whipped body butter (only 4 ingredients). Thecoconutmama.Com. https://thecoconutmama.com/homemade-body-butter

Wills, A. (2019, May 27). 2 great DIY body butter recipes - whipped or unwhipped. Savvyhomemade.Com. https://www.savvyhomemade.com/diy-body-butter-recipes

Comedogenic Ratings List. (2018, April 9). Beneficialbotanicals.Com. https://www.beneficialbotanicals.com/comedogenic-rating

Hale, K. (2021, January 19). Whipped Gingerbread Body Butter. Youbrewmytea.Com.

 https://www.youbrewmytea.com/whipped-gingerbread-body-butter

James, E. (2020, March 11). Is Body Butter Good for Your Face? Ellisjamesdesigns.Com.

https://www.ellisjamesdesigns.com/is-body-butter-good-for-your-face

Marr, K. (2017, March 31). Body butter guide: How to make homemade body butter.

Livesimply.Me. https://livesimply.me/how-to-make-easy-body-butter

Norton, D., MS, & RD. (2014, December 12). Double chocolate DIY body butter.

Backtothebooknutrition.Com.

https://www.backtothebooknutrition.com/diy-double-chocolate-body-butter

Wills, A. (2019a, May 27). 2 great DIY body butter recipes - whipped or unwhipped.

Savvyhomemade.Com. https://www.savvyhomemade.com/diy-body-butter-recipes

Wills, A. (2019b, June 8). A lovely, whipped body butter recipe with raspberry.

Savvyhomemade.Com. https://www.savvyhomemade.com/homemade-whipped-body-butter

Wills, A. (2020, January 26). Winter skin carrot infused body butter recipe.

Savvyhomemade.Com. https://www.savvyhomemade.com/carrot-infused-body-butter

www. facebook.com/senseandserendipityblog. (2017, May 16). DIY Whipped Body Butter for

sensitive skin. Senseandserendipityblog.Com.

https://www.senseandserendipityblog.com/2017/05/diy-whipped-body-butter-sensitive-skin

Bobbie, Tara, Berry, B. W. B., Jeanette, Audrey, Jessica, April, Angela, Jennifer, Maggie,

Marjorie, Monamur, Render, K., Anne-Marie, Angel, Babcock, T., Static, S., Curtell, Berry, A.

W. B., ... LaQuetia. (2011, November 22). Labeling your products : Lip balm. Soapqueen.Com.

http://www.soapqueen.com/bath-and-body-tutorials/lip-products/labeling-your-products-lip-balm

Body Butter Packaging Ideas. (n.d.). Packagingoptionsdirect.Com. Retrieved from

https://packagingoptionsdirect.com/body-butter-packaging-ideas

Bonilla, H. (2017, November 29). The 8 most important FDA regulations for cosmetics

manufacturers. Swktech.Com. https://www.swktech.com/8-important-fda-regulations-cosmetics-personal-care-product-manufacturers/

Fisher, D. (n.d.). How to keep body butter from melting. Thesprucecrafts.Com. Retrieved from https://www.thesprucecrafts.com/keep-body-butter-from-melting-516580

Irvine, D. (2017, July 31). HDPE bottles vs. PET bottles. Raepak.Com.

https://www.raepak.com/hdpe-bottles-vs-pet-bottles

Raychel. (n.d.). 5 tips for preserving homemade & natural body care products.

Mountainroseherbs.Com. Retrieved from https://blog.mountainroseherbs.com/5-tips-preserving-handcrafted-natural-bodycare-products

Tara, Amanda, Berry, B. W. B., Carolyn, Michelle, Brittanie, Anne-Marie, Debbie, Tricia,

Jacqui, lena, carolyn, Holland, J., Allison, Babcock, T., Jay, Mitchell, K., Berry, A. W. B., sisi, ... Rachel. (2011, December 12). How to Label: Lotion. Soapqueen.Com.

https://www.soapqueen.com/bath-and-body-tutorials/lotion/how-to-label-lotion

The best containers for homemade beauty and skincare products. (2021, June 5).

Alifeadjacent.Com. https://alifeadjacent.com/containers-for-diy-beauty-and-skincare-products

Tips for storing your body butter. (n.d.). Simisolanaturals.Com. Retrieved from

https://www.simisolanaturals.com/tips-about-storing-your-body-butter

Wills, D. (2020, February 21). Synthetic & natural preservative for cosmetics & lotions.

Savvyhomemade.Com. https://www.savvyhomemade.com/preservative-for-cosmetics

Clarke, A. (2019, January 30). Shea butter for eczema: Treatment & benefits. Healthline.Com.

https://www.healthline.com/health/shea-butter-for-eczema

Everything you need to know about body butter. (n.d.). Ilovecosmetics.Co.Uk. Retrieved from

https://www.ilovecosmetics.co.uk/blog/everything-you-need-to-know-about-body-butter

Hubbard, A. (2021, May 10). Benefits of body scrubs: Uses, cautions, DIY body scrub recipes. Retrieved from

Healthline.com website:
https://www.healthline.com/health/beauty-skin-care/benefits-of-body-scrubs

How to use body scrubs. (n.d.). Retrieved from
Thebodyshop.com website: https://www.thebodyshop.com/en-ca/tips-and-advice/how-to-use-body-scrub/e/e00070

Types of body scrubs. (2017, August 7). Retrieved from
Healthscopemag.com website:
https://healthscopemag.com/health-scope/types-body-scrubs

Top 8 oatmeal benefits for skin. (n.d.). Retrieved from
100Percentpure.com website:
https://www.100percentpure.com/blogs/feed/top-8-oatmeal-benefits-for-skin

Skin, S. (2018, September 8). Why almond face scrub is one of
the best skin care products for face. Retrieved from Medium
website: https://medium.com/@shaeskin/why-almond-face-scrub-is-one-of-the-best-skin-care-products-for-face-d4d89b742486

Kashyap, T. (2021, April 5). 5 amazing benefits of coffee scrubs
for smooth, clear skin. Retrieved from NDTV Swirlster website:
https://swirlster.ndtv.com/beauty/skincare-5-amazing-benefits-of-coffee-scrubs-for-smooth-clear-skin-2406531

Henry, E. (2018, August 15). Benefits of sugar scrubs for your
skin. Retrieved from Suburbansimplicity.com website:
https://www.suburbansimplicity.com/benefits-sugar-scrubs

Henry, E. (2017, August 21). Benefits of sugar scrubs vs. salt
scrubs. Retrieved from Suburbansimplicity.com website:
https://www.suburbansimplicity.com/benefits-sugar-scrubs-vs-salt-scrubs

Glenn, R. (2019, July 22). Turmeric for skin: 12 benefits and
ways to use it. Retrieved from Greatist.com website:
https://greatist.com/health/turmeric-for-skin

Body scrub ingredients – Matteo essentials. (n.d.). Retrieved from Matteoessentials.com website: https://www.matteoessentials.com/body-scrub-ingredients

10 benefits of botanical body scrubs | Viviane Woodard skincare. (2020). Retrieved from https://vivianewoodard.com/10-benefits-of-botanical-body-scrubs

(N.d.). Retrieved from Ilisagvik.edu website: https://www.ilisagvik.edu/wp-content/uploads/beauty-products-out-of-food.pdf

5 amazing benefits of Sesame Oil for skin. (2018, March 18). Cashkaro.Com. https://cashkaro.com/blog/amazing-benefits-of-sesame-oil-for-skin-uses-its-application/22646

5 ways Olive oil benefits your skin. (2017, August 28). Dermstore.Com. https://www.dermstore.com/blog/olive-oil-benefits-for-skin

6 ways to use Rose essential oil for skin. (2021, June 24). Helloglow.Co. https://helloglow.co/beauty-ingredient-rose-oil

7 benefits of sunflower seed oil for your skin. (n.d.). Bucklersremedy.Com. Retrieved from https://bucklersremedy.com/blogs/the-dirty/7-benefits-of-sunflower-seed-oil-for-your-skin

8 incredible things sunflower seed oil can do for your skin. (n.d.). Pharmagel.Net. Retrieved from https://pharmagel.net/pages/8-incredible-things-sunflower-seed-oil-can-do-for-your-skin

Agarwal, A. (2020, February 14). Here's exactly how you should be using A body scrub. Bebeautiful.In; Be Beautiful India. https://www.bebeautiful.in/all-things-skin/everyday/the-right-way-to-use-a-body-scrub

Allen, M. (n.d.). Ask a dermatologist: Can you use Olive oil for your skin? Byrdie.Com. Retrieved from https://www.byrdie.com/olive-oil-for-skin

Andrea. (2019, January 5). 6 best essential oils for homemade sugar body scrubs. Thebestorganicskincare.Com. https://thebestorganicskincare.com/6-best-essential-oils-for-homemade-sugar-body-scrubs

Aromatherapist, J. L.-C. (2019, May 31). Carrier Oil vs. Essential Oil - A quick guide. Lovingessentialoils.Com. https://www.lovingessentialoils.com/blogs/essential-oil-tips/carrier-oil-vs-essential-oil

Axe, J., DC, DNM, & CN. (2021, October 30). The top uses and benefits of frankincense oil for health. Draxe.Com. https://draxe.com/essential-oils/what-is-frankincense

Bharat, D. (2021, January 6). Beauty care: 5 marvelous benefits of walnut-based products for your skin and hair health. Netmeds. https://www.netmeds.com/health-library/post/beauty-care-5-marvellous-benefits-of-walnut-based-products-for-your-skin-and-hair-health

Carrier Oils - what are Carrier Oils - uses & benefits for skin & hair. (n.d.). Newdirectionsaromatics.Com. Retrieved from https://www.newdirectionsaromatics.com/blog/products/all-about-carrier-oils.html

Herbal Dynamics Beauty. (n.d.). Sweet orange essential oil: Clear skin, clear mind. Herbaldynamicsbeauty.Com. Retrieved from https://www.herbaldynamicsbeauty.com/blogs/herbal-dynamics-beauty/sweet-orange-essential-oil-clear-skin-clear-mind

Isabella. (2020, July 23). Benefits of peppermint Essential Oil for skin care and health I how to use and safety precautions — isabella's clearly. Isabellasclearly.Com; Isabella's Clearly. https://www.isabellasclearly.com/blog/benefits-of-peppermint-essential-oil

Jain, C. (2019, September 10). Walnut oil: 6 must-know benefits that make this oil A skin wonder. Republic World. https://www.republicworld.com/lifestyle/fashion/walnut-oil-6-must-know-benefits-that-make-this-oil-a-skin-wonder.html

Leonard, J. (2018, March 18). 4 olive oil benefits for your face. Medicalnewstoday.Com. https://www.medicalnewstoday.com/articles/321246

Malik, T. (2021a, January 29). Sesame seed oil deserves to be in your beauty closet; here is why. Herzindagi.Com; HerZindagi English. https://www.herzindagi.com/beauty/sesame-seed-oil-beauty-benefits-vitamin-e-acne-scars-article-170381

Malik, T. (2021b, August 4). What is neroli oil and benefits of using it for skin. Herzindagi.Com; HerZindagi English. https://www.herzindagi.com/beauty/neroli-oil-health-benefits-for-skin-article-181379

Marlys, M. (2021, May 27). What to know about carrier oils for skincare. Goodhousekeeping.Com. https://www.goodhousekeeping.com/beauty-products/a36491686/carrier-oils-for-skincare

Miralles, M. (2020, December 2). 5 top Olive oil benefits for the skin. Treurer.Com. https://www.treurer.com/en/blog-olive-oil-culture/health/olive-oil-benefits-for-the-skin

Phototoxic - citrus essential oils and the sun - one essential community. (2016, April 6). Oneessentialcommunity.Com. https://oneessentialcommunity.com/phototoxic-citrus-essential-oils-sun

Rud, M. (n.d.). How to use peppermint oil for soothed, clear skin. Byrdie.Com. Retrieved from https://www.byrdie.com/peppermint-oil-for-skin-4801648

Sesame Oil for Skin - Benefits, Uses & more. (n.d.). Anveya.Com. Retrieved from https://www.anveya.com/blogs/top-tips/sesame-oil-for-skin-benefits-uses-more

Shatzman, C. (2017, November 17). What you need to know about essential oils for pregnancy. Thebump.Com; The Bump. https://www.thebump.com/a/essential-oils-for-pregnancy-basics

Srivastava, K. (2021, April 1). 12 incredible benefits of walnut oil for beauty and health. Bebeautiful.In; Be Beautiful India. https://www.bebeautiful.in/all-things-lifestyle/health-and-wellness/walnut-oil-benefits-for-beauty-and-health

Sunflower oil for skin: 10 benefits, how to use. (n.d.). Fleurandbee.Com. Retrieved from https://fleurandbee.com/blogs/news/sunflower-oil-for-skin

Sunflower oil for skin: Usage, benefits, and tips from beauty experts. (n.d.). Mustelausa.Com. Retrieved from https://www.mustelausa.com/blogs/mustela-mag/sunflower-oil-for-skin

thebirthhour. (2019, April 18). Best essential oils for pregnancy: What to use & avoid [+how to apply]. Thebirthhour.Com. https://thebirthhour.com/essential-oils-for-pregnancy-what-to-use-and-avoid-how-to-apply

TNN. (2014, January 13). 5 beauty benefits of sesame oil. Indiatimes.Com; Times Of India. https://timesofindia.indiatimes.com/life-style/beauty/5-beauty-benefits-of-sesame-oil/articleshow/28466375.cms

Tonelli, L., & Maloney, M. (2019, February 1). These essential oils will work wonders for your skin. Townandcountrymag.Com; Town & Country. https://www.townandcountrymag.com/style/beauty-products/g26011830/best-essential-oils-for-skin

What is the difference between carrier oil and essential oil. (2020, July 9). Pediaa.Com. https://pediaa.com/what-is-the-difference-between-carrier-oil-and-essential-oil

Bly, B. (2019, December 24). DIY Gentle Oat Scrub Recipe. Retrieved from Popshopamerica.com website: https://www.popshopamerica.com/blog/diy-gentle-oat-scrub-recipe

Cinnamon vanilla oatmeal body scrub. (2014, January 13). Retrieved from Mybakingaddiction.com website:

https://www.mybakingaddiction.com/cinnamon-vanilla-body-scrub

Owens, C. (2013, July 26). Homemade coconut oatmeal scrub. Retrieved from Apumpkinandaprincess.com website: https://apumpkinandaprincess.com/homemade-coconut-oatmeal-scrub

Wischnia, B. (2016, January 26). 3 DIY oatmeal scrubs you should make to get your skin glowing. Retrieved from Brit.co website: https://www.brit.co/diy-oatmeal-scrubs

Jin, J. (2019, July 10). Why you need an oatmeal scrub in your life (plus, how to make one easily at home). Retrieved from Purewow.com website: https://www.purewow.com/beauty/diy-oatmeal-scrub

Ives, S. (2019, April 11). Oatmeal benefits for skin. Retrieved from Com.sg website: https://www.stives.com.sg/oatmeal-benefits-for-skin

Lewis, R. (2021, April 28). Oatmeal benefits for the skin: Properties and how to use. Retrieved from Medicalnewstoday.com website: https://www.medicalnewstoday.com/articles/oatmeal-benefits-for-the-skin

Benefits of a Salt scrub massage. (n.d.). Retrieved from Org.uk website: https://www.spaexperience.org.uk/about/blog/benefits-of-a-salt-scrub-massage

Breyer, M. (n.d.). 8 homemade salt and sugar body scrubs. Retrieved from Treehugger.com website: https://www.treehugger.com/homemade-salt-and-sugar-body-scrubs-4858792

MARIN. (2020, November 10). Salt scrub recipes and benefits for skin. Retrieved from Beautycrafter.com website: https://beautycrafter.com/salt-scrub-recipes-and-benefits

Nancy. (2015, January 27). Two Simple DIY Salt Scrub Recipes (you can make!). Retrieved from Artsychicksrule.com website: https://www.artsychicksrule.com/simple-diy-salt-scrub-recipes

What are the benefits of salt scrubs? (2010, June 28). Retrieved from Leaf.tv website: https://www.leaf.tv/5176247/what-are-the-benefits-of-salt-scrubs

Natural beauty: DIY detoxifying sea salt body scrub. (n.d.). Retrieved from Peacefuldumpling.com website: https://www.peacefuldumpling.com/natural-beauty-diy-detoxifying-sea-salt-body-scrub

3 beauty benefits of sugar in your skincare routine - LOOKFANTASTIC. (2018, February 28). Retrieved from Lookfantastic.com website: https://www.lookfantastic.com/blog/discover/3-beauty-benefits-sugar-skincare

DiDonato, J. (n.d.). This is the right way to use a sugar scrub, according to a dermatologist. Retrieved from Byrdie.com website: https://www.byrdie.com/how-to-use-a-sugar-scrub-4771241

Glow sugar scrub (DIY sugar body scrub). (2012, August 27). Retrieved from Simple-veganista.com website: https://simple-veganista.com/diy-edible-sugar-scrub

How to use a sugar scrub: The ultimate guide. (n.d.). Retrieved from Hudabeauty.com website: https://hudabeauty.com/us/en_US/blog-how-to-use-sugar-scrub-55007.html

Irena. (2020, May 3). The best DIY sugar scrub recipes for glowing skin and gift-giving. Retrieved from Countryhillcottage.com website: https://www.countryhillcottage.com/diy-sugar-scrub-recipes

Nguyen, H. (2020, March 6). Top 8 sugar scrub benefits and why you'll love it. Retrieved from Hanaleicompany.com website:

https://www.hanaleicompany.com/blogs/beauty-tips/top-8-sugar-scrub-benefits-and-why-you-ll-love-it

Paris, L. (2021, May 1). Sugar scrubs: Benefits, how to use them, and more - L'oréal Paris. Retrieved from Lorealparisusa.com website: https://www.lorealparisusa.com/beauty-magazine/skin-care/skin-care-essentials/what-is-a-sugar-scrub.aspx

Perry, N. (2014, June 23). Homemade sugar scrub with brown sugar and coconut oil - perry's plate. Retrieved from Perrysplate.com website: https://www.perrysplate.com/2014/06/homemade-body-scrub-brown-sugar.html

Desk, P. (2021, January 8). This DIY Walnut scrub will give you the GLOSSIEST skin ever. Retrieved from PinkVilla website: https://www.pinkvilla.com/fashion/beauty/diy-walnut-scrub-will-give-you-glossiest-skin-ever-591090

DIY rice bran nourishing & exfoliating face mask recipe. (2020, August 12). Retrieved from Womenio.com website: https://www.womenio.com/6226/diy-rice-bran-nourishing-exfoliating-face-mask-recipe

DIY wheat bran and baking soda body scrub. (2016, September 22). Retrieved from Makeupandbeauty.com website: https://makeupandbeauty.com/diy-wheat-bran-and-baking-soda-body-scrub

Honey, A. F. S. (n.d.). Purifying buckwheat facial scrub. Retrieved from Amesfarm.com website: https://www.amesfarm.com/blogs/recipe-box/purifying-buckwheat-facial-scrub

McLintock, K. (n.d.). The average cost of beauty maintenance could put you through Harvard. Retrieved from Byrdie.com website: https://www.byrdie.com/average-cost-of-beauty-maintenance

Moore, C. (2021, March 23). Americans will spend $15G on lifetime skincare, this cosmetics retailer claims. Retrieved from

Fox Business website:
https://www.foxbusiness.com/lifestyle/americans-spend-15g-lifetime-skincare-cosmetics-retailer-claims

Paula's Choice Research & Education Team. (2017, April 14). How omega fatty acids help skin. Retrieved from Paula's Choice website: https://www.paulaschoice.com.au/expert-advice/skincare-advice/ingredient-spotlight/how-omega-fatty-acids-help-skin.html

The WellBeing Team. (2010, October 12). A DIY natural body scrub. Retrieved from Com.au website: https://www.wellbeing.com.au/body/beauty/diy-natural-body-scrub.html

VeganBeautyReview. (2015, September 11). DIY flaxseed scrub [RECIPE]. Retrieved from Veganbeautyreview.com website: https://veganbeautyreview.com/2015/09/diy-flaxseed-scrub.html

8 benefits of facial scrubs & how to use them right. (2021, April 2). Retrieved from Skinkraft.com website: https://skinkraft.com/blogs/articles/benefits-of-facial-scrubs

9 beauty benefits of yogurt for skin & hair - eMediHealth. (2021, May 13). Retrieved from Emedihealth.com website: https://www.emedihealth.com/skin-beauty/yogurt-beauty-benefits

10 amazing coconut milk benefits for hair, face, and skin. (n.d.). Retrieved from Ndtv.com website: https://food.ndtv.com/beauty/10-amazing-coconut-milk-benefits-for-hair-face-and-skin-1421580

Bose, S. (2020, September 4). Benefits of rice water for skin: How to make and use it properly. Retrieved from Bebeautiful.in website: https://www.bebeautiful.in/all-things-skin/everyday/benefits-of-rice-water-for-skin

Don't exfoliate your face with a body scrub — here's why. (n.d.). Retrieved from Skincare.com website: https://www.skincare.com/article/can-you-use-body-scrub-on-your-face

Femina. (2018, January 31). Homemade face scrubs that you need to try right now. Retrieved from Femina.in website: https://www.femina.in/beauty/skin/homemade-natural-face-scrubs-for-healthy-skin-76560.html

Moorhouse, V., & Lukas, E. (2018, January 10). How to exfoliate your dry skin without overdoing it. Retrieved from Instyle.com website: https://www.instyle.com/beauty/how-to-exfoliate-dry-skin

Oatmeal for skin: 10 reasons to add this superfood to your routine. (n.d.). Retrieved from Babobotanicals.com website: https://www.babobotanicals.com/blogs/news/oatmeal-for-skin

Palmer, A. (n.d.). Exfoliation tips to help acne-prone skin. Retrieved from Verywellhealth.com website: https://www.verywellhealth.com/exfoliation-basics-15626

Sehgal, K. (2021, June 1). Olive oil for dry skin: Benefits Of Olive Oil to get moisturized and healthy skin. Retrieved from NDTV Swirlster website: https://swirlster.ndtv.com/beauty/olive-oil-for-dry-skin-benefits-of-olive-oil-to-get-moisturised-and-healthy-skin-2453820

Shunatona, B. (n.d.). Green tea is the superhero ingredient for everything from acne to anti-aging. Retrieved from Byrdie.com website: https://www.byrdie.com/green-tea-for-skin-4843092

Sinha, R. (2013, December 16). 16 best ways to use honey for dry skin. Retrieved from Stylecraze.com website: https://www.stylecraze.com/articles/simple-ways-in-which-honey-can-solve-dry-skin-problems

Wallace, J. (2011). Natural beauty. New Scientist (1971), 209(2796), 27.

(N.d.). Retrieved from Lady-first.me website: https://www.lady-first.me/article/body-and-face-scrub-what-difference,2101.html

4 steps to the perfect DIY body scrub packaging. (2019, August 20). Diysugarscrub.Com.

https://diysugarscrub.com/packaging_design/4-steps-to-the-perfect-diy-body-scrub-packaging

Alphafoodie, S. @. (2018, December 17). DIY coconut oil sugar scrub recipe. Alphafoodie.Com. https://www.alphafoodie.com/coconut-body-scrub

Bonilla, H. (2017, November 29). The 8 most important FDA regulations for cosmetics manufacturers. Swktech.Com. https://www.swktech.com/8-important-fda-regulations-cosmetics-personal-care-product-manufacturers

Homemade body scrub recipes: Make sugar, salt, oatmeal, or coffee scrubs. (n.d.). Homemade-Gifts-Made-Easy.Com. Retrieved from https://www.homemade-gifts-made-easy.com/homemade-body-scrub.html

Raychel. (n.d.). 5 tips for preserving homemade & natural body care products. Mountainroseherbs.Com. Retrieved from https://blog.mountainroseherbs.com/5-tips-preserving-handcrafted-natural-bodycare-products

Rohde, E. (2021, April 13). Sugar scrub labels - 11 reasons why you need them for your products. Yourboxsolution.Com. https://www.yourboxsolution.com/blog/sugar-scrub-labels

Body Scrub Products Market - global industry analysis, current trends, and forecast by 2026. (n.d.). Retrieved from Transparencymarketresearch.com website: https://www.transparencymarketresearch.com/body-scrub-products-market.html

Hubbard, A. (2021, May 10). Benefits of body scrubs: Uses, cautions, DIY body scrub recipes. Retrieved from Healthline.com website: https://www.healthline.com/health/beauty-skin-care/benefits-of-body-scrubs

Made in the USA
Las Vegas, NV
21 December 2024

15150184R00266